WHAT
DO WHEN
THE DOCTOR
SAYS IT'S

Asthma

WHAT TO DO WHEN THE DOCTOR SAYS IT'S

Asthma

Everything You Need to Know About
Medicines, Allergies, Food, and Exercise
to Breathe More Easily Every Day

PAUL HANNAWAY, M.D.

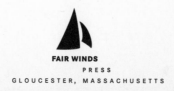

FAIR WINDS
PRESS
GLOUCESTER, MASSACHUSETTS

Text © 2004 by Paul Hannaway, M.D.

First published in the USA in 2004 by
Fair Winds Press
33 Commercial Street
Gloucester, MA 01930

08 07 06 05 04   1 2 3 4 5

ISBN 1-59233-104-1

Library of Congress Cataloging-in-Publication Data available

Cover design by Laura Shaw Design
Book design by *tabula rasa* graphic design

Printed and bound in Canada

The information in this book is for educational purposes only.
It is not intended to replace the advice of a physician or medical
practitioner. Please see your health-care provider before beginning
any new health program.

To my patients and families afflicted with asthma

CONTENTS

Acknowledgments

I would like to thank the following individuals for their contributions to this manuscript: Rachel Butler, Carlene Roundy, Marilyn Nagle, Dr. Albert Sheffer, and my wife Bunny for her thoughtful input and wonderful illustrations.

About the Author

Dr. Hannaway, an asthma sufferer and father of two asthmatic children, offers a unique perspective on asthma. Over the past three decades he has treated thousands of patients with asthma and has authored numerous publications, including the American Medical Writers Award-winning, *The Asthma Self-Help Book*. Dr. Hannaway, a fellow of the American Academy of Allergy, Asthma & Immunology, and the American College of Allergy, Asthma and Immunology, is an Assistant Clinical Professor at Tufts University School of Medicine.

CHAPTER ONE

The Emerging Epidemic

Most, if not all, of the developed countries in the world have experienced a dramatic increase in the incidence of asthma. My own experience with asthma verifies that developed countries are in the midst of an asthma-allergy epidemic. As a child and young adult, I was the only kid on the block who suffered from asthma. I don't recall any other friends, classmates, or teammates in grade school, high school, or college who were rushed to the local emergency room or the school health center for acute asthma treatment or needed to puff on an asthma inhaler before or after athletic events.

This picture has changed dramatically. Over the past twenty years, two of my five children and scores of their friends have developed asthma. Parents who attend any type of sporting event will see an incredible number of participants puffing on an asthma inhaler. While the true incidence of asthma in the United States during the 1950s and early 1960s is not well documented, trends indicate that the number of asthma sufferers has probably increased tenfold since the 1950s. I cannot think of any other chronic disease with such alarming numbers.

In 1980, it was estimated that 6.8 million Americans had asthma. According to the National Center for Health Statistics, the number of asthmatics increased to nearly 18 million cases in the United States in 2004. The number of asthma deaths has also increased threefold, from 1,674 deaths in 1977 to over 5,000 fatalities in 2002. Deaths from asthma in the five- to fourteen-year-old age group have doubled in the past fifteen years. An alarming study by the Johns Hopkins School of Public Health estimates that the number of people afflicted with asthma and the number of asthma deaths will double in the next decade. If these figures are correct, 29 million Americans will have asthma, and ten thousand will die from their disease in the year 2010.

The increase in asthma is most dramatic in children under age five, where the number of cases has tripled since 1980. There are a half-million new cases of childhood asthma in the United States every year. Six million youngsters under the age of eighteen now have asthma. California, New York, and Texas, the most populated states, have the most cases of asthma. Each year the CDC (Centers for Disease Control) collects information about the incidence of chronic diseases like asthma by random telephone surveys of over 250,000 homes in all fifty states and four U.S. territories. The 2002 survey found nearly 12 percent of respondents were told by a health professional that they had asthma. The lowest prevalence was found in South Dakota (8.6%) and the highest in Puerto Rico (19.6%). The highest rates of asthma were found in whites (7.6%), blacks (9.3%), and multiracial (non-Hispanic) groups (15.6%). The levels of asthma prevalence were higher in 2002 than they were in 2001 and 2000. The one bright spot in this report found that the number of asthma deaths had leveled off after 1996.

This increase in asthma cases coincides with an across-the-board rise in all types of allergic diseases, including allergic rhinitis or hay fever, atopic dermatitis or eczema, and food allergies. A survey from the American College of Allergy, Asthma and Immunology (ACAAI) found that allergies were twice as prevalent as previously believed.

Nearly 40 percent of all Americans now suffer from some type of allergic disease.

In 2004, the New England Asthma Regional Council assessed the incidence of asthma in that six-state region and found more than four hundred thousand children had been diagnosed with asthma. Children from the poorest families were almost twice as likely to have asthma, especially in black or Hispanic families, where the attack rate was 50 percent higher than whites. Across the region 12 percent of children had asthma. In Massachusetts alone, nearly 185,000 children had asthma.

The Inner-City Epidemic

The asthma epidemic has hit American inner cities the hardest. Inner-city dwellers, especially minority children and young adults, have experienced an explosive increase in asthma cases. There are twice as many asthma cases in the heavily industrialized northeast than in sparsely populated rural Western states like South Dakota. The poorer sections of New York City have been hit the hardest. The rate of hospitalization for asthma in the Bronx and Harlem is twenty times higher than asthma admissions in the more affluent boroughs of the Big Apple. A New York City study of 1,319 children in East Harlem elementary schools found an astounding asthma prevalence rate of 35 percent. This area has a high percentage of Puerto Rican families who may be more genetically predisposed to asthma, especially if brought up in a dwelling infested with rats, mice, cockroaches, or smoking parents. Similar patterns were found in a Philadelphia survey of nine thousand children attending eighty public schools.

Inner-city blacks and Hispanics have a disproportionately high rate of asthma-related emergency room visits and hospitalizations. These unfortunate minorities are four times more likely to die from asthma. Genetic and ethnic patterns might be the reason for this inner-city epidemic; minorities' high exposure to outdoor air pollutants, dust mites, cockroaches, smokers, and animal allergens, especially from cats and rodents, is also a factor. In other words, the genes load the asthma gun and the environment pulls the trigger.

Air pollution, especially ozone and diesel particles, may also be big players in this scenario. A University of California study found more asthma in high ozone areas where children played outdoor sports after school versus children living in low ozone areas. European research centers find more asthma in residents of homes close to major motorways.

Some asthma experts believe inner-city children spend too much time indoors. An inner-city asthma study funded by the National Institutes of Health found that only 40 percent of inner-city children played outside after school hours, because of the potential threat of neighborhood violence. The asthma epidemic is not localized to inner cities. A substantial, although less dramatic, increase in asthma cases has been observed in suburban populations. This brings up an important question: Why are we experiencing a rise in asthma cases and an increase in the rate of asthma hospitalizations and asthma deaths, when we have much more effective drugs to treat asthma than we did twenty years ago?

The Impact of the Asthma Epidemic

This emerging asthma epidemic severely impacts health-care costs and the quality of life for asthma sufferers. Asthma is the leading chronic disease among children, accounting for ten million lost school days. Asthma is the third leading cause of hospitalization for children under age fifteen. Next to upper respiratory infections, asthma is the leading cause of school absenteeism. The number of office visits for asthma has gone from 4.6 million per year in 1980 to over 10 million per year in the late 1990s.

In the year 2000, the price of asthma has nearly tripled to 18 million dollars. When you add the cost of office visits, emergency room care, and hospitalizations to the increasing prices of asthma drugs, the economic burden of asthma care in the United States approaches $20 billion per year. Asthma-care costs now exceed the combined total costs of AIDS and tuberculosis.

In a survey of 401 adults with asthma in Northern California, the total cost per patient for asthma care totaled $4,912. The largest cost component was asthma drugs at $1,605 per patient. Those with mild disease cost less—$2,646 per year versus those with severe disease—$12,813 per year. Eighty percent of all the money spent on asthma care is spent on 20 percent of all asthmatics. This "80-20 rule" applies to a lot of other chronic diseases like diabetes and congestive heart failure. There are nearly six hundred thousand emergency room visits per year for childhood asthma. Hospitalizations account for more than half of all these expenses. In children under age four, hospitalizations eat up more than three-fourths of all childhood asthma costs. Thus, considerable savings would occur if hospitalizations were reduced, especially if you have more severe asthma.

What about the effect of asthma on one's quality of life? A Philadelphia survey found 27 percent of asthmatics were awakened with asthma at least once a week. One in every three asthmatics missed school or work, and nearly half agreed that asthma interfered with exercise or daily activities. One in every three Philadelphia asthma sufferers made an unscheduled visit to their doctor or clinic in the past year because of their disease. Forty-two percent required a hospitalization or an emergency room visit in the past year. Disturbed sleep from nocturnal asthma led to decreased productivity from the working parent(s) and poor academic performance by the student with asthma. How many of these people were seeing an asthma specialist on a regular basis? The survey found that only 50 percent of people with mild asthma had ever seen an asthma specialist, and one-third of people with severe asthma had never seen a specialist. The final conclusions of this Philadelphia study were that most asthmatics had an impaired quality of life and were not receiving proper specialty asthma care.

The Worldwide Epidemic

Ireland, England, Scotland, New Zealand, and Australia have all reported an increase in the frequency and severity of asthma. The European epidemic is most pronounced in the United Kingdom and lowest in Eastern European countries like Albania. The World Health Organization estimates that there are 150 million asthmatics in the world, and 180,000 people die each year from asthma. This represents a 50-percent increase in worldwide asthma deaths in the past decade.

In 1828, Dr. John Bostok noted that hay fever was more common in "the upper middle classes of society, some indeed of high rank." A similar experience was reported in the U.S. in the nineteenth century when George Miller Beard deemed hay fever to be "a rare disease found only in the privileged classes of New York City—in male professionals, literary and businessmen, and rarely noted in those who till the soil." The overall increase in allergic diseases in the second half of the twentieth century was more commonly seen in "thin middle-class children of above average intelligence."

The better the economy of a country, the more asthma. The lowest rate is found in Southeast Europe—Albania and Romania. There is more asthma in Japan (13 percent) versus Indonesia (2 percent). In South and Central American countries like Brazil and Costa Rica, the prevalence of asthma is between 20 and 30 percent of the general population. The incidence of asthma in the Western Pacific Region varies from 50 percent in the Caroline Islands to virtually zero asthma cases in New Guinea. Statistical trends clearly show that the emerging asthma-allergy epidemic is taking place in more developed countries. The most startling study on asthma prevalence comes from New Zealand where a long-term followup of asthmatic children born in 1972–1973 found that 27 percent still had asthma twenty-five years later. Persistent adult asthma was more common in women, dust-mite-allergic children, and smokers. Many of these children who developed asthma at an early age had significant airway obstruction by nine years of age.

CHAPTER TWO

Why Asthma?

Taking a Closer Look at the Normal Lung

Think of your lungs as two big pouches of air containing millions of smaller sacs connected to tubes. Another way to look at the lung is to picture it as an upside-down tree, in which the tree trunk is the trachea or windpipe, the largest branches are the main bronchial tubes, the smaller branches are the bronchioles, and the leaves are the air sacs or alveoli. The primary function of our lungs is to inhale oxygen-rich air and to remove or exhale the body's waste gas—carbon dioxide. This all-important exchange of oxygen and carbon dioxide takes place deep in our lungs, in tiny air sacs called alveoli. Before air reaches these air sacs, it must pass through the trachea, or windpipe, that divides into the right and left bronchial tubes that in turn connect to the right and left lungs. These main bronchial tubes then further subdivide into smaller tubes called bronchioles on the way to the air sacs.

Once air enters the alveoli, inhaled oxygen crosses into the blood stream and is then transported to the heart, which pumps life-sustaining oxygen to all parts of the body. A separate network of blood vessels brings the body's waste gas, carbon dioxide, back to the alveoli, before it is removed from the body when you exhale.

The Asthmatic Lung

What goes wrong in the asthmatic lung? First, let us look at the walls of the bronchial tubes. These walls are made up of various cells, muscle tissue, and mucus-secreting glands. In the normal lung, air moves in and out of the alveoli and bronchial tubes, and your lungs maintain a perfect balance of oxygen and carbon dioxide throughout your entire body. In asthma, the bronchial tubes are abnormal. They are constantly inflamed or swollen, and air movement is blocked. The bronchial tubes are lined by tens of thousands of cells, including white blood cells and specialized cells called mast cells, which are loaded with toxic chemicals called mediators. These mast cells release their chemicals, causing the walls of the bronchial tubes to swell up and become inflamed. The end result of a swollen and obstructed bronchial tube: you will have shortness of breath, coughing, and wheezing—the three cardinal symptoms of asthma.

Think of your bronchial tubes as a garden hose. When the hose is open, water flow is unimpeded, but if you pinch or bend the hose, the flow of water is obstructed, and the obstructed hose produces a hissing or wheezing sound. In asthma, this bronchial obstruction can often be reversed, and the bronchial tubes can return to a normal state. Thus, one older medical definition of asthma is "reversible obstructive airways disease," often abbreviated as ROAD. Two other more catchy names for asthma are "twitchy lung syndrome" and "wheezy bronchitis." It is now recognized that tissue inflammation in the bronchial tubes is the major cause of chronic asthma.

The Inflammation Theory

The rediscovery of an old concept has dramatically altered the way asthma specialists treat asthma. In 1873, Sir Charles Blackley demonstrated that hay fever and asthma sufferers challenged with an allergen did not begin to sneeze or wheeze until several hours after inhaling the allergen, and sometimes their sneezing and wheezing lasted several days after the allergen was removed. In 1952, Karl

Herxheimer expanded these observations when he reported two very distinct components to an inhaled allergen. He called these components the early phase asthma response and the late phase asthma response. Additional studies have shown that asthmatics react in two ways to inhalation challenges, both in real life and in the laboratory.

The coughing and wheezing that develops within minutes, peaks in thirty minutes, and resolves in one to three hours is called the early phase asthma response. The wheezing that starts three to four hours after an inhalation challenge, peaks in four to eight hours, and lasts twenty-four to seventy-two hours is called the late phase asthma response. This late phase response that causes chronic inflammation of the bronchial tubes is the most important feature of chronic asthma. This important finding produced dramatic changes in asthma therapy, as it has been shown that asthma drugs have different actions in the early and late asthma responses.

The asthma-relieving or bronchodilating drugs like the beta-agonist drugs, theophylline, and the anticholinergic drugs open up or dilate the bronchial tubes. For this reason, they are called relievers or bronchodilators. These drugs prevent or relieve the symptoms of the early response, but have little or no effect on the late phase inflammatory response. On the other hand, anti-inflammatory medications such as the cromolyn-like drugs, the cortisone drugs, and the new leukotriene modifiers will not relieve asthma symptoms once they occur, but they prevent or control the late phase or inflammatory response. Such drugs are called controllers or anti-inflammatory drugs. How should these findings be applied to the real world of asthma therapy? The clinical implication is obvious. As we shall see, every patient with persistent asthma requires both a relieving and a controlling asthma drug.

What Causes Inflammation?

There is no simple answer to this question. No one group of cells or chemical mediators fully explains asthma. It is best to think of asthma as a symphonic orchestra where the end point of inflammation is the result of many sections of instruments—the cells and chemical mediators. Once this immune orchestra starts to play, the bronchial tube becomes swollen and inflamed. In 1989, I described asthma as a reversible obstructive airways disease, or ROAD. This older asthma definition meant that lung functions could be reversed or improved with treatment. This was wrong. Lung function may never return to the normal range in some people with severe asthma, even with ideal treatment. The newer definition of asthma depicts it as a chronic disorder of the airways in which many inflammatory cells play a role. In susceptible individuals this inflammation causes recurrent wheezing, chest tightness, and coughing, especially at night or in the early morning. Symptoms are usually associated with an airflow limitation that usually reverses with treatment. The inflammation also causes an increase in airway responsiveness to a variety of stimuli that asthma researchers call bronchial hyperreactivity.

Remodeling—A New Concept

Studies have shown that many nonsmoking asthmatics suffer from low lung function similar to chronic lung disease, such as bronchitis or emphysema. In some cases, this loss of lung function is permanent. This discovery has led to a new asthma term called "airway remodeling." What do asthma researchers mean when they talk about airway remodeling? Remodeling is the buzzword used to describe permanent structural damage to the airway in asthma. I like to think of airway remodeling as a scarring reaction to chronic inflammation and the loss of the ability to repair or reverse lung inflammation. When the bronchial tubes remain chronically inflamed, they overreact or become hyperreactive to all types of irritants or inhaled particles and aeroallergens. When airway inflammation persists, the bronchial tubes may become permanently scarred. Fortunately, remodeling or scarring is not a common occurrence, but it does explain why many asthmatics who have never smoked have low lung functions.

Asthma specialists know the greatest loss in lung function in asthma occurs within three years after the onset of asthma symptoms. This loss in lung function may occur as early as six or seven years of age in asthmatic children. The concept of airway remodeling has promoted several important questions. Would early and aggressive use of the inhaled cortisone drugs, especially in young children, prevent remodeling? Preliminary studies show that young children with persistent asthma who were treated with inhaled cortisone drugs for three years had better lung function than those children treated with only bronchodilating drugs. Children who delayed starting inhaled cortisone for two to three years after the onset of their asthma had lower lung functions than children started on inhaled cortisone right after their asthma was first diagnosed. This loss in lung function occurs even more rapidly in adult-onset asthma.

Remodeling can be a factor in young children, many of whom are not diagnosed as having asthma until several years after the onset of coughing and wheezing. In my opinion, early and aggressive anti-inflammatory therapy in this age group may prevent chronic asthma in adulthood, whereas a delay in diagnosis and lack of proper therapy may lead to lung remodeling and severe debilitating asthma later on in life.

Now that we have reviewed what goes wrong in the asthmatic lung, you might now ask: why asthma? While there is no correct answer to this compelling question, the bottom line is that you can place most of the blame on your parents or grandparents. Your ancestors are guilty of passing on an asthma gene or genes, or your parents may have kept too clean a home or not allowed you to play in the dirt during infancy or early childhood. As we shall discuss in detail, asthma and other allergic diseases are a result of a complex interaction between your genetic background, your immune system, and environmental exposures. In other words, your genes load the gun and the interaction between your immune system and environment pulls the trigger.

Those Elusive Asthma Genes

What are genes? Every living organism, including all plant and animal life, contains a substance called deoxyribonucleic acid, more commonly known as DNA. Human DNA is composed of nearly thirty thousand genes that act like computer chips that program your body to develop individual characteristics such as baldness, brown hair, or blue eyes. DNA that is passed down from one generation to another also determines what diseases you may or may not develop during your lifetime. Asthma is labeled as a complex genetic disease. That means that there are several genes that predispose one to develop asthma, and they interact in a complex manner. In genetic language this means that asthma is due to several family traits or genes which, when combined with the right (or wrong) environmental exposures, may lead to clinical disease. The inheritable component of asthma and other allergic diseases has long been recognized, due to clusters of asthma and allergic diseases in families and identical twins.

Not all individuals who inherit an asthma or allergy gene will develop asthma or an allergic disease. This is called non-penetrance. Penetrance refers to those individuals with a certain gene who do develop the disease state. In a complex genetic disease, like asthma, penetrance is never complete. This explains why asthma may skip generations. Other diseases that have a similar genetic makeup include diabetes, cancer, and heart disease. This contrasts to cystic fibrosis that is transmitted by a single dominant gene. Either you have cystic fibrosis or you don't, and environmental exposures play no role.

The results of the United States Human Genome Project, started in 1990, are now unfolding. This project has found that about thirty thousand human genes program the three billion DNA building blocks that underlie all human biology. The full sequencing of human DNA will result in the identification of the two to three hundred thousand proteins that are used to make up a human being. This new era in genetic research will lead to new ways to diagnose and treat allergies and asthma, and have a profound impact on all inherited diseases.

Additional research has found an abnormal gene in people experiencing near-fatal or fatal asthma attacks. Genes not only determine if and when you get asthma; they also program the severity level of your asthma. Once a specific asthma gene (or genes) is found, the proteins produced by the gene can be identified. Some of these gene proteins are "good proteins" that prevent one from developing asthma. Other proteins are "bad proteins" that trigger a genetic disease like asthma. Genetic researchers will someday develop chemicals to block the bad proteins and stimulate the good proteins and therefore prevent the development of inherited diseases.

The ABC's of the Immune System

In the early part of the twentieth century, asthma was thought to be a purely psychosomatic disorder. One famous victim of this foolish concept was President Theodore Roosevelt. Leading psychiatrists of the day theorized that Roosevelt's asthma was the result of an unstable home and a domineering father. But Roosevelt's asthma improved dramatically when he left his eastern home to live in Wyoming. His recovery was undoubtedly due to a combination of growth, vigorous exercise, and breathing the clean Wyoming outdoor air. Eventually these erroneous psychiatric concepts would give way to a more plausible explanation of asthma that focuses on man's most important body system—the immune system.

Humans are equipped with a powerful biological defense, or immune system, made up of a complicated network of organs, cells, and glands that defend and protect or confer immunity against all kinds of foreign invaders. The four major components of our immune system are our bone marrow, thymus gland, spleen, and lymph nodes or glands.

These organs produce a variety of blood cells, chemicals, and protective proteins including antibodies, whose main purpose is to defend against or ward off outside invaders. Such invaders include viruses, bacteria, parasites, allergens, and a host of other stimuli, including cancer-inducing substances. When our immune system fails to work properly, we get sick. The failure of our immune system to protect us from an outside invader ranges from a simple virus that triggers the common cold to the deadly Acquired Immune Deficiency Syndrome or AIDS virus. AIDS is the most blatant example of what happens to man when his immune system fails to defend itself against outside invaders. The two basic components of the immune system are the humoral system and the cell-mediated immune system.

The Humoral Immune System

Before discussing humoral immunity, we must define the difference between an antigen and an antibody. A foreign substance, such as a virus or allergen, that enters the body is called an antigen. When the body's immune system encounters an antigen, certain white blood cells called B-cells make a protective protein against the antigen. This protein is called an antibody. The next time your body encounters this antigen, the protective antibody will kill or neutralize the antigen. When the immune system is functioning normally, you develop immunity to invading antigens that lasts for years or even a lifetime. This is the basis of all vaccines or immunizations. The immune system can be programmed to induce permanent immunity or protection by injection or vaccination with foreign proteins (antigens) derived from viruses and bacteria.

An ideal example of humoral immunity centers on childhood vaccines. In infancy and early childhood, vaccines are administered to children to protect them against common diseases like polio, measles, mumps, diphtheria, and chicken pox. After vaccination, the immune system manufactures protective antibodies against these vaccines. Later on, when you are exposed to the natural virus or bacteria, the immune system will kill or neutralize the virus or bacteria. The end result is that you do not get these once-common childhood diseases.

During our lifetime, we produce tens of thousands of antibodies that protect us from all types of infections, parasites, and diseases, thereby allowing us to lead a normal, healthy life. However, sometimes the immune system overreacts to an antigen, and we may develop an autoimmune disease like lupus or rheumatoid arthritis. In some individuals the B-cells overreact to harmless allergens in our environment and start making too much allergic antibody. As we shall see, asthma and other allergic diseases are the direct result of an overreaction of our immune system to normally harmless outside invaders or antigens.

Cell-Mediated Immunity

The second component of our immune response is called cell-mediated immunity. In cell-mediated immunity, antigens or invaders are processed by a series of cells in the immune system called T-cells. They are called T-cells because they are derived from the thymus gland. These T-cells are present in your lymph nodes or glands. Once an antigen reaches the lymph gland, several types of T-cells come into play. Some T-cells kill the infected cells (killer T-cells), some suppress the antigen (suppressor T-cells), and some actually help combat the antigen (helper T-cells). The T-cells are even more important to our discussion than the antibody-producing B-cells, as it is the T-cells and their products that determine whether or not you will develop asthma and/or other allergic diseases.

The Allergic Reaction

Throughout our lifetime, the humoral side of the immune system manufactures thousands of antibodies or immunoglobulins each time we are exposed to viruses, bacteria, parasites, or allergens. These immunoglobulins (abbreviated Ig) are divided into five groups: IgA, IgD, IgG, IgM, and IgE. The immunoglobulin most involved in protecting us against common viruses and bacteria is the IgG antibody, commonly known as gammaglobulin antibody. The all-important immunoglobulin that plays the major role in asthma and allergic diseases is called immunoglobulin E, or IgE antibody. Approximately one in every five individuals inherits an asthma-allergy gene (or genes) that primes their immune system to overproduce this allergic or IgE antibody. The fascinating aspect about allergic or IgE antibody is that it protects people against common tropical and parasitic diseases. Through the process of evolution and diminished exposure to worms and parasites, this once-friendly IgE antibody has turned on mankind. It is now a "bad-boy antibody" that overreacts to common environmental allergens such as dust mites, molds, animal parts, foods, drugs, insect stings, and innocuous pollen grains. The 40 million unfortunate Americans who have inherited the tendency to overproduce IgE antibodies are more likely to develop allergic conditions like asthma, hay fever, eczema, or a food or drug allergy.

The Mast Cell and IgE Antibody: A Match Made in Hell

What makes the IgE antibody so influential in asthma and other allergic conditions? Unfortunately, IgE antibody has a special affinity for one of the more important cells in the human body, called the mast cell. Millions of mast cells line your skin, nose, intestines, and bronchial tubes. Each mast cell contains more than a thousand tiny granules that are loaded with dozens of potent chemicals or mediators. These mediators range from the oldest and most widely known chemical, called histamine, to the newly discovered group of mediators—the leukotrienes. In essence the IgE antibody attaches itself to the mast cell, which is a chemically laden bomb just waiting to explode. When you inherit the capacity to become allergic and make IgE antibodies, the first time you are exposed to a potential allergen like ragweed pollen, you do not get hay fever. However, after repeated exposures, your immune system's B-cells produce IgE antibodies to the ragweed pollen. These IgE antibodies then attach themselves to the surface of the mast cell. The next time you inhale ragweed pollen, it binds to the

IgE antibody sitting on the surface of the mast cell. This combination of antigen (like ragweed pollen) and IgE antibody triggers a chemical reaction in the mast cell that releases its powerful mediators, like histamine, into the surrounding tissues. The surrounding tissues then get very inflamed and swollen. When the mast cell erupts in your nose, you sneeze; when the lungs are targeted, you wheeze; and if the skin is the site of the reaction, you itch. The end result of this mast cell eruption is the classical SWI, or sneeze, wheeze, and itch reaction that typifies allergies. (You may be interested to know that as a former baseball-softball player, I sponsor a softball team in my local town called the SWISOX. Just like my beloved Boston Red Sox, I am still waiting for them to win it all.)

Common aeroallergens that trigger this SWI reaction include dust mites, molds, animals, pollens, stinging insects, foods, and drugs. When doctors first discovered that allergens could induce attacks of hay fever, asthma, or hives, they set out to develop ways to determine if a person was allergic or sensitive to these substances. Thus, the specialty of allergy was born, and the allergist became the doctor who could isolate and identify specific allergens that caused people to sneeze, wheeze, or itch. Over the past three decades, advances in immunology have produced a greater understanding of our immune system. Such discoveries are beginning to explain the potential reasons for the asthma-allergy epidemic, and define why allergen exposures during pregnancy and early infancy may alter the way our immune system handles allergens for the rest of our lives. Let's take a closer look at how our immune system handles foreign invaders or antigens.

Antigens enter our bodies through various portals, including our skin, nose, lungs, and gastrointestinal tract. Since we are mainly concerned with asthma, let us explore what happens when we inhale a foreign antigen like a virus, bacteria, or allergen into our lungs. After an antigen or allergen is inhaled, it settles on the lining of the lung, a region called the mucosal surface. The body's first attempt to defend itself against the inhaled antigen is the production of mucus by glands known as mucus glands. We all know that when we get a cold or breathe in any kind of foreign substance like an air pollutant, the lining of our respiratory tree produces excess mucus, or phlegm, called mucin. Mucus does not kill or de-activate a virus, bacteria, or allergen, but simply wraps it up in a coating of gel. This mucus is then coughed up, spit out, or swallowed and destroyed in the intestinal tract. When this mucin system is operating normally, we protect ourselves from inhaled viruses, bacteria, air pollutants, or allergens.

However, when the invader evades this mucus trap, it crosses the surface of the mucosa, where it is met by a class of cells called DC or dendritic cells—biology students will remember them as the macrophages. This cell then ingests the invading antigen and breaks it up into smaller particles called peptides. The DC cell then acts like a taxicab that transports the peptides to nearby lymph nodes or glands where the critical phase of the immune response takes place.

When Lymph Glands Attack

One of the major components of our immune system is the network of lymph nodes or glands located throughout our body. These glands essentially act as filters against invading agents, by mounting an immune response to neutralize the invading antigen while at the same time avoiding local tissue injury. This response explains why you get swollen glands in your neck when you experience a strep throat. This lymph node reaction involves the interaction of dozens of various cells and chemicals. As we discussed earlier, the two most important cells involved in the immune response are the B-cells and the T-cells. The B-cells make antibodies like allergic or IgE antibody, and gammaglobulin or IgG antibody.

The T-cells are more complicated. T-cells that kill the invader are called killer T-cells. Other T-cells that suppress an invader are labeled suppressor T-cells. Lastly, the helper T-cells program various other pathways in the immune system. The helper T-cells send out signals that bring other cells into the area to combat the invader. These helper T-cells are labeled Th (h is for helper) cells, and are the most influential of all the T-cells, as they determine the path the immune system travels after being exposed to an outside invader or antigen. Helper or Th cells can be divided into two major cell types labeled the Th1 and Th2 cells. These all-important Th1 and Th2 immune cells determine if you do or do not develop asthma or other allergic diseases.

When the Th1 cells are activated, they release chemicals called cytokines that drive the immune system away from an allergic response to an invading allergen. Too much Th1 cell activity may lead to autoimmune diseases. On the other hand, the Th2 cells are pro-allergic cells. They produce cytokines that signal the B-cells to manufacture allergic-IgE antibody. The Th2 cells also send out signals to attract allergy blood cells like the eosinophils, basophils, and mast cells from other parts of the body. The cells that heed the call of the Th2 cells migrate into the local area of antigen invasion and secrete mediators like histamine and leukotrienes into the surrounding tissues. Once these chemicals hit the local tissues, they cause swelling and inflammation.

Again, the site of the reaction determines if you will sneeze, wheeze, or itch. Thus, the allergic reaction is the end result of those all-important Th2 cells driving the immune response in the direction of an inflammatory or pro-allergic response. Doctors can indirectly measure Th2 cell activity by measuring the level of allergy blood cells (eosinophils) and IgE antibody in your serum. Individuals with allergic or atopic conditions like asthma, hay fever, and eczema have high levels of eosinophils and IgE antibody.

Crunching the Numbers: Th1 versus Th2

What drives our immune system in either of these two directions? Genes or hereditary factors play a big role, as asthma-allergy genetic codes passed from one generation to the next send the immune system down the Th2 allergy highway. People who do not carry an allergy-asthma gene are more likely to mount a Th1 or non-allergic response to an invading allergen. The second factor that determines what road your immune system takes is your environmental exposure. The reason some individuals who carry an asthma-allergy gene never develop asthma or other allergic diseases is that they had little or no exposure to allergy-triggering antigens such as foods, animal allergens, dust mite, molds, and pollens at key periods of their lives. On the other hand, those who have inherited the asthma-allergy gene may have no chance if they are exposed to an offending allergen at a certain time in their lives.

What is the right or wrong time? Immunologists now believe that allergen exposures during pregnancy, early infancy, and childhood are the key factors. The most fascinating aspect of the recent discoveries in this immune scenario is that a pro-allergy or Th2 response may be determined by what your mother eats, inhales, or rubs on her body during pregnancy, or by what you are exposed to or injected with in infancy or early childhood. As we shall discuss later, whether or not your immune system travels down the Th2 allergy highway may even be determined by the size of your family, your month of birth, attendance at a day-care center, or early exposure to farm animals or household pets.

The developing fetus usually has markedly different blood and tissue types from the mother. All unborn babies are essentially a mass of foreign protein living in their mother's womb. Transplant immunology has taught us that when you try to graft or unite different types of organs or blood types, the host or recipient will promptly reject the graft or organ transplant. This is called the graft-versus-host reaction. One of the miracles of the animal kingdom is that a fetus or unborn infant is rarely rejected by the mother's immune system. The reason for the mother's acceptance of this foreign organism is that the mother turns off her Th1 response in pregnancy and the unborn baby mounts a strong Th2 immune response that prevents rejection by the host mother.

Thus, all healthy infants are born with a pro-allergic Th2 immune system. Why don't all newborns then follow the allergy-prone Th2 highway? Here's where Mother Nature takes over. In newborns destined to be non-allergic, the immune system shifts over to the non-allergic Th1 pathway shortly after birth. If a newborn swallows harmless bacteria during a vaginal delivery, the Th1 response is turned on. Just the opposite occurs in infants born with an asthma or allergy genetic makeup. When the fetus or newborn carrying the asthma-allergy gene is exposed to a variety of antigens or allergens early in life, or possibly even in utero, the end result is that the pro-allergy or Th2 system remains in control. Let's take this one step further. What has happened in the last twenty years that favors the Th2 pathway and the onset of the asthma-allergy epidemic?

The asthma-allergy epidemic has taken place in less than a generation—too short a time to be blamed on genetic or evolutionary factors. The answer to the epidemic may lie in changes in our environment and lifestyle. Alterations in maternal and infant eating habits, a rise in deliveries by Cesarean sections, environmental exposures (or lack thereof), and the expanded use of childhood vaccines and antibiotics may keep the Th2 system operating. A pro-allergic Th2 response then sends the infant or young child down the allergy highway. Allergy researchers like to use the term "allergic march" to describe those infants who go on to hit for the cycle and develop all of the "big four" allergic conditions—eczema, food allergy, allergic rhinitis (hay fever), and asthma.

CHAPTER THREE

How Doctors Diagnose Asthma

Asthma is usually not a very difficult disease to diagnose. The major symptoms of asthma are coughing, wheezing, shortness of breath, and chest tightness. These symptoms are quite variable and are often triggered by the common cold; viral respiratory infections; vigorous exercise, especially in cold air; exposure to allergens when dusting or vacuuming; and exposure to household pets. Other common triggers include pollens, foods, chemicals, and air pollutants. Symptoms often interfere with sleep. Wheezing is the cardinal symptom of asthma, and in one study of people with a variety of heart and lung disorders, wheezing was named as their major symptom by more than 90 percent of people with asthma.

Your Medical History

What happens during your first visit to a doctor or health-care provider when asthma is suspected? First and foremost, the health-care provider should take a detailed medical history, often with the aid of a written questionnaire. You will be asked to describe your symptoms, when they began, what makes them better or worse, and what medications relieve symptoms. He or she will inquire about seasonal patterns, smoking habits, effects of exercise or cold air, and exposure to polluted air. The pattern of symptoms provides important clues. Seasonal flare-ups suggest pollen allergy, whereas year-round symptoms are more common with dust mite, cockroach, and animal allergy. Nocturnal or early morning symptoms suggest allergen exposure in the bedroom—dust mites in a mattress or feathers and molds in a pillow. Headaches, nocturnal cough, throat clearing, or foul breath may signal a chronic sinus condition. Frequent heartburn and indigestion suggests the presence of gastroesophageal reflux disease, or GERD. The doctor should inquire whether you have any other conditions closely associated with asthma, such as hay fever, eczema, or allergic reactions to foods or drugs. He or she will want to know if you have repeated bouts of ear or sinus infections, nosebleeds, or a loss of smell or taste.

A detailed environmental history focuses on potential asthma triggers in your home, school, or workplace. It should cover the age and location of the home, the type of heat and air-conditioning system, the presence of a fireplace or wood-burning stove, whether there is a basement, the use of central or room humidifiers and/or air conditioners, and the proximity of nearby industry or sources of air pollution. The doctor will probably ask you to describe whether the home is damp, and report present or past water damage.

Additional questions should focus on the patient's bedroom, including the location of the bedroom, whether pets are allowed in the room, the type of pillow and mattress, and whether dust mite-impermeable covers are used on the pillow, mattress, and box spring. The doctor should inquire about the presence of dust catchers such as stuffed animals, wall-to-wall carpeting, upholstered furniture, books, and drapes. Further history should include questions about the school or work environment, and any other locations where the patient spends a significant amount of time. The doctor should also review the results of any previous treatment or tests, including skin tests, blood tests, and X-ray studies.

Getting Physical

The next step in your office visit is the physical examination, which will focus on your skin, eyes, ears, nose, throat, and chest. The doctor will look at your skin for signs of eczema or hives. Inflammation in your eyes may signify an underlying eye allergy or allergic conjunctivitis. Dark circles under the eyes, called "allergic shiners," or swelling in the nose are both telltale signs of allergic rhinitis or hay fever, commonly associated with asthma. The chest exam is the most important part of the physical examination. The doctor will rely on the stethoscope to detect wheezing and gauge the rate of air movement in and out of your chest. The doctor may ask you to take a deep breath or briefly exercise to make it easier to detect wheezing. An astute asthma doctor can often diagnose asthma by just looking at a patient's chest and observing what is called the barrel-chest deformity. When people with chronic asthma constantly use their chest and rib muscles to move air in and out of their lungs, their chest wall is stretched to the limit, and it expands, giving the chest a barrel-like shape. In an asymptomatic patient, however, the physical examination may be completely normal. In those cases, the history will yield critical information.

Step into the Lab

The next part of the evaluation involves laboratory testing. Commonly performed tests include a nasal or a sputum smear, where mucus from the nose or chest is examined under a microscope in the search for an excess amount of eosinophils, the telltale allergy blood cell. Eosinophils are the hallmark of asthma or an ongoing allergic reaction, and are increased in numbers in asthma and allergic diseases. Eosinophils usually comprise 3 to 4 percent of all white blood cells in your body. The level of eosinophils in your body, measured by a blood test called the total eosinophil count, often parallels the severity of asthma. Other diagnostic tests the doctor may order include a sweat test to rule out the possibility of cystic fibrosis, serum immunoglobulins to rule out an immunodeficiency disease, a sinus CAT scan to check for underlying sinus disease and intraesophageal pH monitoring or a barium swallow study to determine the presence of gastroesophageal reflux disease or GERD.

The IgE Test

One important blood test is the serum IgE test, which measures the amount of allergic or IgE antibody in your body. IgE levels increase slowly till age ten to fifteen then slowly decline with age. A high IgE level indicates that allergies may be playing an important role in your asthma. This test often predicts if an infant or a young child will ever develop asthma or allergies, as the IgE level may be elevated years before asthma or hay fever symptoms begin. A study of health and development in 562 children in New Zealand by Dr. Malcolm Sears disclosed that young boys had more asthma than girls, and the prevalence of asthma was directly related to the serum IgE level. No asthma was found in children with IgE levels less than thirty-two units, whereas more than one-third of those with high IgE levels had asthma. The higher the IgE level, the greater the chance that the child had asthma. Although a high serum IgE level is often seen in the allergic or asthmatic patient, a normal IgE level does not rule out allergy. Likewise, a high IgE level does not always predict allergic asthma.

Breathing Tests

Pulmonary function studies, called spirometry or lung function tests, are breathing tests that measure your lung capacity. In a breathing test, you breathe into a closed tube connected to a machine which measures how much air you can expel from your lungs in one single breath (lung capacity) and how fast you can expel it. The key measurement in asthma is the amount of air you blow out in one second. This is called the FeV1, or one-second vital capacity. Measurement of the FeV1 is a more sensitive way to detect airway obstruction than the clinical history or the physical examination. Many people are "poor perceivers" of their asthma symptoms. This means they are unable to sense airway obstruction until their lungs are functioning at a very low level. Thus, lung function tests should be done in all people when the diagnosis of asthma is suspected. The assessment of lung function helps to determine the severity of the asthma and outline an asthma treatment program. When the first set of breathing tests are abnormal, you may be asked to inhale a quick-acting bronchodilator drug and repeat the breathing test. If the second test shows more than a 10 to 15 percent improvement in the FeV1, the diagnosis of asthma is almost a certainty. Follow-up measurements of lung function are the best ways to monitor the response to asthma therapy.

Machines that measure lung function range from relatively inexpensive devices or spirometers to sophisticated high-tech computerized equipment that records all facets of lung function. Any doctor who treats persistent asthma should use some sort of spirometer machine to diagnose and follow the progress of people with asthma. The NIH asthma guidelines state "spirometry is the gold standard for the diagnosis and management of asthma." One new inhalation test that will vastly help to diagnose asthma is the inhaled nitrous oxide test. Nitrous oxide or NO is a gas we all normally exhale. However, if our lungs are inflamed, as in asthma, the level of exhaled NO is high. This test, not yet available for general use, simply involves blowing up a balloon, attaching it to an NO analyzer and measuring the amount of NO in your expired air.

The Peak Flow Meter

It is now possible for people with asthma to measure their own lung functions at home, school, or work with small, inexpensive, portable pulmonary function devices called peak flow meters. These peak flow meters measure how fast you can expel air from your lungs. They are very helpful in detecting the early stages of an asthma relapse, and determining if substances in the home, school, or workplace are triggering asthma. The peak flow meter plays a pivotal role in helping people adhere to the new asthma guidelines' step-up and step-down approach to asthma drug therapy.

Allergy Skin Tests

When the medical history, physical exam, or blood tests suggest that allergens may be triggering asthma, skin testing is indicated. What are skin tests? In 1873, Dr. Charles Blackley discovered the cause of his own hay fever when he scratched a small amount of grass pollen on his skin and produced a small hive-like reaction at the test site. Amazingly, basic skin test techniques have changed very little since Blackley's important century-old observation.

There are three basic types of skin tests: the prick or puncture, scratch, and intradermal test. In the prick test, the test antigen or allergen is placed on top of the skin, and the skin is pricked through the drop. In a scratch test, the skin is lightly scratched, and a drop of the test allergen is placed onto the scratched area. The weaker scratch or prick tests are done first, to minimize the chances of triggering a dangerous allergic reaction.

When the scratch or prick tests are negative, a stronger intradermal test is administered. In the intradermal test, allergen is injected beneath the skin with a very small needle. When you have an allergic or IgE antibody to the test allergen, the antigen combines with the IgE antibody and a wheal and flare reaction or a hive will develop at the test site. The flare refers to the redness, and the wheal is the white center in the middle of the redness. The size of the skin test often reflects your level of sensitivity to the allergen.

The older scratch test method, often a traumatic experience, especially for young children, has been replaced by the prick test method, where several allergens can be tested at the same time. One such method, called the Multi-Test, allows a panel of several allergens to be lightly placed on the skin at one time with little or no discomfort or pain to the patient. Skin tests help identify allergies to inhaled substances like dust mites, molds, pollens, and animals. A competent allergist can determine if allergens are playing a role in your asthma by performing fifty to sixty skin tests in one or two office visits. In younger children you can often get by with ten to twenty tests.

Despite their ancient origins, skin tests are a quick and accurate way to determine the presence of allergy. As the clinical history is a poor predictor of skin test reactivity, I perform skin tests in all new patients with asthma. They are relatively inexpensive on a cost-per-test basis, and are very safe when carried out under the supervision of a knowledgeable physician experienced in allergy skin testing.

Allergy Blood Tests

It is also possible to detect allergies with a blood test known as the radioallergosorbant or RAST test. In this test a small sample of your blood is processed through an analyzer to see if your blood contains allergic or IgE antibodies to a specific allergen. RAST tests are very helpful when the doctor cannot perform skin tests because of skin eruptions or undue fear of needles or if there is a chance of inducing an allergic reaction with the skin test, as may be the case in severe peanut or tree nut allergies. While allergy blood tests are helpful, they have three major disadvantages. They are not quite as accurate as skin tests, they are ten times more expensive, and the results are not immediately available.

An allergy specialist will interpret your skin and blood tests and correlate these with your clinical history. A positive test does not mean that you are having symptoms to the test substance at the time of testing, as skin tests may be positive years before symptoms begin or remain positive long after allergy symptoms have subsided.

X-ray Studies

A chest X-ray should be obtained in all people with recurrent respiratory symptoms in order to rule out rare lung diseases and other potential causes of airway obstruction such as congenital defects or foreign bodies. The chest X-ray findings in asthma may vary from normal to an overinflated lung with scattered areas of atelectasis or a collapsed lung. Chest X-ray findings may support the diagnosis of asthma in a child who is too young to perform lung function tests. Given the close association between asthma and sinusitis, a sinus X-ray should be considered in people who have a history of persistent rhinitis, nocturnal coughing, headaches, or asthma that is difficult to control. In very young children, plain sinus X-rays may suffice. In older children and adults a limited sinus CAT scan has proven to be a better way to diagnosis chronic sinus disease.

Calling in the Specialist

The early symptoms of asthma—chest congestion, coughing, and wheezing—usually first come to the attention of the pediatrician, internist, or family doctor. Many primary care physicians are quite capable of treating mild or even moderate asthma. However, when asthma complicates a patient's lifestyle by interfering with school or work, limiting exercise, or causing frequent visits to the doctor's office or emergency room, the expertise of an asthma specialist may be required. Two types of doctors are experts in the care of asthma, the allergist-immunologist and the lung specialist or pulmonologist. These doctors have taken two to three additional years of training after completing a three-year residency in either pediatrics or internal medicine. The pulmonologist treats diseases like asthma, emphysema, bronchitis, and tuberculosis, while the allergist specializes in the care of allergic or atopic diseases like asthma, hay fever, food or drug allergy, and allergic skin disorders.

Once you and/or your primary care provider decides you need to see an asthma specialist, you must choose between these two types of doctors. The asthma-allergy specialist is best at diagnosing and treating asthma when there is an allergic component to asthma or the patient has other allergic conditions. Pulmonologists are experts in managing people with severe asthma, especially if they have coexisting pulmonary diseases like bronchitis or emphysema or have required repeated hospitalization or intensive care for asthma relapses. I frequently co-manage these people with severe asthma. In this situation I take care of the patient outside of the hospital, while the pulmonary-intensive care specialist takes over when the patient requires hospitalized care.

The Advantages of Specialty Care

Numerous studies provide strong support for specialty care for people with complicated asthma who are at risk for emergency room visits or asthma hospitalizations. Doctors Michael Mellon and Robert Zeiger from the Kaiser-Permanente Medical Center in San Diego, California, found a marked reduction in nighttime wheezing, asthma relapses, and emergency room visits in people referred to an asthma specialist when compared to people who did not receive specialty care. Intensive outpatient asthma treatment programs, staffed by medical personnel skilled in the delivery of asthma care, improve outcomes and asthma control. Specialty care should be a two-way street. The asthma specialist does not usually need to take over total control of the patient, but should work closely with the primary care provider. Some people only need to be seen by the specialist once or twice a year, at which time the asthma specialist quarterbacks the patient's asthma program. Such follow-up visits should include a letter to the primary care provider, who in turn can monitor a patient's progress and ensure compliance with the recommendations of the asthma specialist.

I prefer to evaluate new patients with asthma in two or three visits. Once the diagnosis of asthma has been established during the first visit, my nursing staff and I will present an asthma education plan to the patient or family. Such a program incorporates educational videos, asthma literature, an asthma action plan, and hands-on instruction in the use of the peak flow meters and asthma inhalers. Implementation of the asthma action plan is extremely important. A detailed review of environmental controls is essential if you have a documented allergy to indoor and outdoor aeroallergens. Between visits, you must monitor lung function with a peak flow meter. During the summary visit, the doctor should review the results of lab tests, breathing tests, skin tests, medication programs, peak flow readings, and he or she should answer any questions you might have.

After the summary visit is concluded, I dictate a report for the referring or primary care physician and the patient or family. This report can then serve as a reference source for both the primary care provider and the patient or family when a review of the asthma action plan or treatment program is necessary. Such a report is especially helpful when a patient is away at school or is traveling and has to visit a hospital or doctor unfamiliar with the patient's clinical history and treatment program. In my summary report, I classify asthma into one of

THE 1997 NHLBI REPORT

The 1997 report divided asthma into four groups on the basis of symptoms and peak flow readings:

- Mild intermittent asthma: fewer than three episodes per week, fewer than three nocturnal asthma attacks per month, and normal peak flow readings between episodes.
- Mild persistent asthma: symptoms more than twice a week, but not every day, nighttime asthma more than twice a month, and variability in peak flow rates.
- Moderate persistent asthma: daily asthma requiring rescue beta-agonist drugs, nighttime asthma more than once a week, and up to a 30-percent decrease in peak flow readings.
- Severe persistent asthma: continual asthma which limits activities, frequent nighttime asthma, and peak flows less than 60 percent of normal readings.

the four new categories proposed by the new NHLBI Guidelines: mild intermittent asthma, mild persistent asthma, moderate persistent asthma, and severe persistent asthma.

A Closer Look at Managed Care

In my first twenty years of practice, most complicated cases of persistent asthma were referred to asthma specialists for evaluation. People with mild to moderate asthma were usually co-managed by the primary care provider and the asthma specialist. More severe or difficult-to-manage asthma was closely followed by the asthma specialist. This pattern of asthma care dramatically changed once managed care medicine entered the health-care arena in the 1990s. In an effort to reduce costs, managed care organizations and insurers began limiting patient access to specialists. Managed care programs encouraged primary care providers to treat a wide variety of complicated illnesses, including asthma, diabetes, arthritis, and cardiovascular and skin diseases. In some tightly managed care organizations, primary care physicians are economically penalized when they refer too many patients to specialists. No one will debate the fact that the "gatekeeper approach" has reduced the costs of medical care, at least in the short term.

In turn, specialty doctors and national organizations were asked to provide treatment guidelines to primary care doctors for many chronic diseases, including asthma. When one considers the vast array of asthma medications now available for the treatment of asthma, even asthma specialists, like myself, have difficulty keeping current and finding the right combination of asthma medications necessary to control a difficult patient with persistent asthma. The key to managing any chronic disease is patient education, which requires time on the part of the health-care provider.

Today, the time of an average visit to a primary care provider is seven minutes. Thus, while overworked primary care practitioners may have the knowledge and a proper set of guidelines at their disposal, they may not have the time to properly educate and care for patients and families with chronic asthma. One telephone survey of 12,385 primary care physicians found that one in every four physicians felt that the scope of care that they were asked to provide was greater than it should be.

Patients, families, employers, and insurers recognize the value of specialty care. American health-care consumers are rebelling against gatekeeper-rationed care. The pendulum has swung back to easier access to specialty care. Many primary care physicians I deal with have embraced this trend in care, as they were not enthralled with insurers that forced them to care for sicker patients without specialty input.

One study of 28,000 asthma patients in five managed care plans around the United States found that asthma patients treated by specialists had 37 percent fewer hospitalizations and 55 percent fewer emergency visits than patients treated by primary care physicians. Thus, specialty asthma care actually saved money for the insurance companies. Asthma patients treated by specialists were more likely to be using inhaled anti-inflammatory drugs and less likely to need rescue medications, which means that their asthma was under better control.

Guidelines for Specialty Care
What are the current guidelines for the need to see an asthma specialist? The NIH expert panel report on asthma recommends specialty referral in the following situations:

- Difficulty maintaining control of asthma
- Frequent emergency room visits or life-threatening attacks
- Inability to meet the goals of care set by the primary care physician after three to six months of therapy
- Symptoms that are unusual or difficult to diagnose
- Severe hay fever or sinus disease
- Asthma requiring intense asthma education
- Candidates for allergy injections

- Severe asthma requiring high-dose inhaled or oral cortisone (prednisone)
- Need for more than two bursts of oral cortisone in one year
- Young children with moderate to severe asthma who require daily long-term asthma therapy

The key element to reducing asthma-related health-care costs is teaching patients and caretakers to identify asthma triggers, know the early warning signs of asthma, and develop asthma action plans that will reduce the need for expensive emergency visits or hospitalizations. One of the major ways to reduce asthma costs is to identify asthma sufferers at an earlier age. While asthma is a chronic condition, it is quite different from most other chronic diseases in that it starts early in life. Proper asthma care in infancy or early childhood may prevent the development of lifelong asthma.

CHAPTER FOUR

Diseases Associated with Asthma

Your genetic makeup, and the environmental exposures that drive your immune system down the asthma highway, may also induce other allergic diseases, such as allergic rhinitis (hay fever), atopic dermatitis (eczema), and food and drug allergy. Two other diseases commonly associated with asthma that do not require the presence of asthma-allergy genes or environmental exposures to allergens are chronic sinus disease and gastroesophageal reflux disease, or GERD.

One Airway—One Disease

Over the past three decades, most allergy specialists tended to separate allergic rhinitis and asthma and consider them as two distinct conditions. Now there is convincing evidence that they are one disease entity. The belief is that these two conditions are part of a "united inflamed airway." The buzzword is "one airway—one disease." Most people with asthma (80 percent) have allergic rhinitis and 25 to 50 percent of people with allergic rhinitis have asthma. In one European Health Survey, three thousand Swedish respondents with allergic rhinitis had five times more asthma than the rest of the population. Another survey found that 60 percent of Swedish schoolchildren with asthma also suffered from allergic rhinitis. Studies have shown that when these two conditions coexist in the same patient, symptoms are worse than when a patient has only allergic rhinitis or asthma.

Allergic Rhinitis

Allergic rhinitis, commonly called hay fever, is a relative newcomer to the allergy stage. While the ancient Greeks described asthma and food allergy, there is no reference to hay fever until the tenth century, when Persian scholar Rhazes described the causes of the coryza that took place in the spring when roses were in bloom. In the early twentieth century, hay fever was considered to be a rare illness of the upper class. The Scottish doctor and golfer John Morrison Smith described his own hay fever while still in medical school:

"I gradually recognized that it was not an ordinary cold and that the symptoms were much worse on the golf course or even during a nice day rowing on Loch Lomond. At first I did not know what I had, and neither did any other doctor I encountered in the next two or three years..."

Just 100 years later, millions of people now have hay fever or allergic rhinitis. The hygiene hypothesis is one possible reason for this meteoric rise in the prevalence of allergic rhinitis. While nearly 18 million Americans have asthma, more than twice as many—approximately 40 million people—suffer from allergic rhinitis. The prevalence of allergic rhinitis has followed the rise in asthma cases; like asthma the incidence of allergic rhinitis has tripled over the past twenty years in most developed countries.

There are two forms of allergic rhinitis—seasonal and perennial. Seasonal hay fever is caused by exposure to tree, grass, or weed pollens. Perennial, or year-round allergic rhinitis, is triggered by exposure to dust mites, molds, and animal parts. Some authorities believe that untreated allergic rhinitis leads to asthma. This concept has been difficult to prove, as there are few well-researched population studies that have followed individuals with allergic rhinitis for several years. Two decades ago, Dr. Guy

Settipane identified a group of freshman students at Brown University in Providence, Rhode Island, who had allergic rhinitis and positive allergy skin tests. Dr. Guy Settipane tracked these Ivy League students for twenty years after their graduation. Twenty years after graduation, 10 percent of the students with allergic rhinitis had developed asthma.

In a similar study in Italy, 40 percent of more than five hundred students with allergic rhinitis developed asthma within eight years of follow-up. I used to believe that allergic rhinitis, even if untreated, did not cause asthma but simply preceded it. Now I am not so sure. This concept raises an interesting question. Would aggressive treatment of allergic rhinitis, including administering immunotherapy or allergy injections, especially to young children, prevent the development of asthma? Several worldwide studies now underway should ultimately answer this very important question.

The major symptoms of allergic rhinitis are sneezing, itchy nose and eyes, and clear, watery discharge. People with seasonal hay fever report symptoms during specific pollen seasons, while those with year-round or perennial allergic rhinitis complain when house dust mites, molds, and household pets precipitate or aggravate their symptoms.

People who suffer from long-standing allergic rhinitis, especially children, can often be diagnosed just by looking at their facial characteristics and mannerisms. There is often a discoloration and swelling under the eyes called "allergic shiners." When nasal obstruction persists, the typical open-mouth or adenoidal face is apparent. Frequent rubbing of an itchy nose results in the allergic salute, which produces a transverse "allergic crease" across the lower third of the nose. In allergic rhinitis, the mucus membranes inside the nose are often pale-bluish in color, as opposed to the typical red color seen in non-allergic rhinitis or the common cold. The treatment of allergic rhinitis includes antihistamines, decongestants, and anti-inflammatory nasal sprays similar to those used in asthma, combined with proper environmental controls. In more persistent cases, allergy injections or immunotherapy may be indicated.

Atopic Dermatitis

Some babies develop an itchy skin condition known as eczema or atopic dermatitis. This is the first sign that a child has inherited the dreaded asthma-allergy gene. Eczema is a chronic skin disorder closely linked with asthma, allergic rhinitis, and food allergies. When eczema develops before three months of age, the risk of developing food and inhalant allergies and asthma is significantly increased. Seventy-five percent of children with eczema at age three months will become allergic to inhalants by age five. Eczema is often accompanied with allergen sensitization and a high IgE allergic antibody level. Population studies have found that, like asthma and allergic rhinitis, the incidence of eczema has tripled over the past two decades. In some developed countries, eczema now strikes one in every ten infants. Skin biopsies have demonstrated that eczema is a complex disorder involving many of the same inflammatory cells seen in asthma. Major eczema triggers include foods, aeroallergens, and bacterial products. The symptoms of eczema include an itchy patchy skin eruption on the face, arms, or legs, especially in the folds of the elbows and knees. As much of the skin eruption in eczema is self-induced by a scratching patient, doctors have labeled eczema as "the itch that rashes."

Conventional eczema treatment includes antihistamines to relieve itching, topical cortisone creams to control inflammation, and antibiotics when secondary infection is present. Additional local measures include avoidance of irritants, dietary elimination of proven food allergens, skin hydration, and skin moisturizers. Recent clinical trials have found new immunomodulating (non-cortisone) agents, like tacrolimus (Protopic) and picrolimus (Elidel), to be very beneficial in eczema treatment. Eczema is often the first step in the "atopic march" where infants first develop eczema, then food allergies, and later on in childhood they suffer allergic rhinitis or hay fever and asthma. These unfortunate children who have "hit for the cycle" will experience all of the big four allergic conditions: eczema, food allergy, hay fever, and asthma. Present-day research is now focusing on more aggressive ways to treat eczema in early infancy and possibly block this "atopic march" in early childhood.

Chronic Sinus Disease

Chronic sinus disease is undoubtedly one of the most neglected diseases of our time. The more accurate medical term for chronic sinusitis is now chronic rhinosinusitis as most cases of sinusitis are accompanied by nasal symptoms or rhinitis. Figures from the United States Department of Public Health indicate approximately 31 million Americans have sinus disease, causing one hundred thousand lost days from school and work. Chronic rhinosinusitis can be an important trigger of asthma in both children and adults, and its presence should be ruled out in any difficult-to-control asthma patient.

Our sinuses are four paired air cavities surrounding the nose. Each sinus has a small opening, called an ostium, which allows secretions from the sinus cavity to drain into the nose. The varied functions of the sinuses include their role in smell and taste, voice quality, and production of mucus. They also make our heads much lighter. If we did not have air-filled sinus cavities, our head would be as heavy as a bowling ball. The linings of your sinuses contain many glands, which secrete mucus. Your sinuses propel this mucus into your nose with the help of hair-like structures called cilia. Mucus flow removes harmful particles like viruses, bacteria, pollutants, and allergens. When the movement of mucus out of the sinus is blocked, mucus backs up and the sinus cavity becomes fertile ground for bacterial overgrowth. Sinus infections, therefore, most commonly accompany or follow a viral respiratory infection or the common cold. Predisposing factors to sinus infections include allergic rhinitis, deviation of the nasal septum (the bone between the two sides of the nose), nasal fractures, nasal polyps, cigarette smoke, and pressure changes from flying, swimming, and diving. Another new type of sinusitis is called allergic fungal sinusitis where the nasal discharge is very thick: like peanut butter. This form of sinus disease is more likely to be found in people with asthma and aspirin allergy. Rarer illnesses that cause chronic rhinosinusitis include immune deficiency disorders and cystic fibrosis.

Several mechanisms have been proposed to explain why sinus infections trigger asthma. Sinus inflammation may be transmitted to the lung by nerve reflexes connecting the upper and lower respiratory airway. Other experts argue that the asthma symptoms associated with sinus infections are a result of aspiration of mucus and postnasal drip into the lung. Finally, there is an emerging school of thought that chronic rhinosinusitis disease and asthma may be one single disease syndrome that is triggered by inflammation in both the lower and upper respiratory tract. This theory is supported by the fact that the same inflammatory cells are present in the asthmatic lung and in swollen sinus cavities.

The symptoms of an acute sinus infection are readily apparent. People complain of headache or pain and tenderness over the cheeks or above the eyes. They have a yellow-greenish or purulent nasal discharge and a constant cough. More subtle symptoms of chronic disease include fatigue, nasal stuffiness, and postnasal drip that may or may not be associated with a loss of smell and taste. Another common complaint in difficult-to-diagnosis sinusitis, especially in children, is foul breath—or as one mother aptly put it, a "dragon breath" odor. Pediatricians used to think that sinus infections were rare events in infants and toddlers, as it was assumed that their sinus cavities were not very well developed. This has been shown to be untrue, as infants and young children do have sinus cavities that can easily become infected at any age.

If your asthma is difficult to control, you should be evaluated for sinus disease. The diagnosis is made by taking a careful history, physical examination, and X-ray studies. While plain sinus X-rays may be helpful in young children, in most cases plain sinus X-rays are useless and a sinus CAT scan is needed. Part of the difficulty in making the clinical diagnosis of sinusitis is that the signs and symptoms of the disease often overlap with many common childhood respiratory disorders, including the common cold or allergic rhinitis. Two features that distinguish sinusitis from viral upper respiratory infections are the length and severity of the symptoms. In allergic rhinitis, the nasal discharge is usually watery or clear in color. Nasal congestion, cough, and a thick yellow-green nasal discharge that lasts longer than ten days increase the likelihood of a chronic sinus infection.

How to Treat Sinus Disease
Your sinusitis can be treated with systemic decongestants, mucus thinners, topical cortisone sprays, and nasal washings with salt water. Drink plenty of fluid to thin out the thick mucus that may be blocking the narrow sinus openings. Antibiotics are essential in treating sinus infections. Sometimes it may be necessary to treat a sinus infection with antibiotics for four to six weeks. People who have several sinus infections a year that do not respond to appropriate medical management should be evaluated for potential sinus surgery. New, sophisticated surgical techniques, such as endoscopic sinus surgery, offer hope to people with chronic or refractory sinus disease. Results with the newer high-tech sinus surgical procedures are much better compared to older, more primitive and invasive sinus surgery.

In a study at the UCLA School of Medicine, forty-eight children with bad sinus disease and asthma were aggressively treated for their sinus disease. After five weeks of treatment, thirty-eight of these children stopped wheezing and were able to discontinue all their asthma medicine. Similar results were observed in adult studies in Washington, D.C., and St. Louis, although adults were more likely to require surgery to control sinus disease.

The important point about all these sinus studies is that individuals with asthma and coexisting sinus disease may be completely unaware that they have sinusitis. Their symptoms may only include a mild post-nasal drip or a nagging cough. I have seen many people with "silent sinus disease," whose only complaint was bad breath in the morning. Astute doctors should closely question their patients about sinus symptoms and obtain a sinus CAT scan when they suspect the presence of hidden sinus disease. Remember, if you have asthma you are three to five times more likely to have chronic rhinosinusitis disease!

Gastroesophageal Reflux Disease

Ingested foods and beverages are transported to the stomach and the rest of the intestinal tract by the esophagus or food pipe. The junction between the esophagus and stomach is guarded by a muscle or sphincter that prevents food and stomach acid from being regurgitated back up into the esophagus. However, in some individuals this sphincter does not completely close, and food and stomach acid flow back up or reflux into the esophagus or the back of the throat, resulting in indigestion and heartburn. Anyone who has overindulged in a fancy restaurant has experienced reflux. When reflux symptoms persist on a regular basis, the condition is called gastroesophageal reflux disease or GERD. An emerging theory now proposes that reflux of stomach contents may predispose one to sinus disease when stomach contents are refluxed into the back of the throat and into the sinus cavities. This new syndrome is called supraesophageal reflux disease or SERD.

Approximately 60 million Americans have GERD. Asthma specialists have long suspected that there was a strong link between reflux and asthma. Reflux symptoms are nearly twice as common in people with asthma. Several studies found that nearly 50 percent of people with asthma suffered from acid reflux that could trigger asthma symptoms. Many of the people in these studies (65 percent) had "silent reflux" and denied having any reflux symptoms whatsoever. Why are asthmatics more prone to reflux symptoms? They may have a nervous system abnormality that reduces the pressure gradient between their esophagus and stomach and allows stomach acid to easily reflux back up the esophagus. Overreaction by the diaphragm—the large muscle that separates the chest cavity from the abdomen—may also promote reflux.

While it is now well established that asthmatics have more reflux than non-asthmatic patients, it is still not clear if reflux triggers asthma or if asthma triggers reflux. The literature on this issue is conflicting. If reflux triggers asthma, adequate control of reflux should improve asthma symptoms. Many clinical trials show modest improvement in asthma symptoms, but little or no improvement in lung functions with anti-reflux therapy. Such treatment includes antacids, antihistamine drugs that block the release of stomach acid, and drugs called proton pump inhibitors or PPIs that lower the production of stomach acid. Dietary and lifestyle restrictions in reflux therapy include avoiding fatty and acidic foods, minimizing caffeine and alcohol intake, eating smaller meals, not eating before bedtime, and elevating the head of one's bed.

People with severe reflux who do not respond to aggressive medical management may require a surgical procedure, called fundoplication, where the muscle between the esophagus and stomach is tightened by placing a band around it. The results of reflux surgery are difficult to evaluate, as most studies have serious design flaws. University of Washington researchers studied ninety patients with reflux who were randomly assigned to receive the anti-ulcer drug cimetidine, a placebo drug, or undergo reflux surgery. After six months, all three groups had fewer asthma symptoms, particularly those who received cimetidine and surgery. When cimetidine was discontinued, many people relapsed. Over a long-term follow-up period, the surgically treated group improved the most. This and other studies imply that reflux plays a significant role in asthma and doctors should not ignore the co-existence of heartburn and indigestion in people with asthma.

Anyone who suffers from moderate or persistent asthma should be considered a potential reflux victim, especially if they complain of heartburn, frequent burping, indigestion, or coughing and wheezing during or after eating. Reflux is difficult to diagnose because so many people have asymptomatic or "silent" reflux, which requires special diagnostic tests. Such tests require the insertion of a tube into the esophagus to measure the amount of acid regurgitated back up into the esophagus. This is called pH monitoring. A special X-ray study, called a barium swallow, involves the swallowing of a radioactive dye to see if the dye is refluxed from the stomach back up into the esophagus.

When confronted with an asthmatic with suspected reflux, it may make more sense to initiate a trial of anti-reflux therapy rather than immediately ordering a pH study or a barium swallow. Most GERD experts advise putting people suspected of having GERD or SERD on a three-month trial of a PPI drug before resorting to invasive tests. A recent seminar I attended on GERD made two very important points about the PPI drugs: PPIs are often underdosed and they do not work well when taken on an empty stomach. PPI drugs should be taken thirty to forty-five minutes before your biggest meal of the day, which for most people is their dinner meal. The five PPI drugs available in the U.S. are Prilosec, Prevacid, Aciphex, Protonix, and Nexium.

CHAPTER FIVE

Common Asthma Triggers

Many people believe asthma is only triggered by exposure to aeroallergens. This is a total misconception, as there are hundreds of potential asthma triggers, including: indoor and outdoor aeroallergens, irritant chemicals and air pollutants, beverages and food products, viral and bacterial infections, and adverse psychosocial factors (Table 5.1).

Aeroallergens

The best understood of all asthma triggers are the aeroallergens in our indoor and outdoor air that set off an allergen-antibody reaction when inhaled into your nose or lung. Aeroallergens, such as house dust mites, feathers, molds, insect parts, pollens, and animal allergens, have several common characteristics. They must be small and light enough to remain airborne over long periods of time, and a brief exposure to tiny amounts of allergen will induce symptoms in sensitized individuals. Airborne allergens can be found anywhere—indoors, outdoors, at home, at work, or at school. Pollen and mold allergens fluctuate with the seasons, while perennial allergens such as house dust mites, cockroaches, and animal allergens can be present in our indoor air on a year-round basis.

TABLE 5.1. TEN COMMON ASTHMA TRIGGERS

- Aeroallergens
- House dust mites
- Cockroaches, rodents
- Molds
- Pollens
- Animal allergens
- Air pollutants
- Chemicals and foodstuffs
- Viral and bacterial infections
- Psychosocial factors

House Dust Mites

House dust has been recognized as an important asthma trigger for centuries. Indoor dust is not quite the same as outdoor dust. Outdoor dust or just plain dirt is a simple non-specific irritant. Indoor house dust is an incredibly complex mixture of dust mites, cotton fibers, cellulose, mattress parts, animal hairs, mold spores, dead insects, discarded food particles, and bacteria. Seventy percent of all allergic asthmatics are sensitive to house dust, and for many it is their only significant allergy.

Dust allergic asthmatics usually cough or wheeze shortly after arising in the morning, or during the dust season, which in northern climates coincides with the heating season—late fall to early spring. Warm, heated indoor air creates turbulent air currents throughout the home that increase the circulation of dust particles. Dust levels tend to be much higher in older homes, damp homes, basement apartments, and in carpeted dwellings heated with forced-hot-air systems.

In 1964, two Dutch scientists, Drs. Spieksma and Voorhorst, startled the world of allergy research when they discovered that a microscopic-sized arthropod of the Arachnid insect family, the house dust mite, was the major allergen in house dust. Dust mites are tiny, sightless, eight-legged insects that look like creatures from a late-night horror film. Unlike their spider and tick cousins, they are not visible to the naked eye, and they do not bite or transmit any diseases. What is even more frightening than the mite's appearance is its living and eating habits. House dust mites live in bedding, carpets, upholstery, and other textiles, where they feed on skin scales, fungi, bacteria, and various human secretions. There are thousands of different species of mites, but so far only a few are known to cause allergic reactions. One species, *D. farinae,* does well in prolonged dry weather, while the other major allergy-inducing mite species, *D. pteronyssinus,* thrives in damp, humid environments.

The dust mite's favorite snack is your very own human skin scales. Mites are no dummies. To get closer to their cherished food supply, mites congregate in mattresses, rugs, and stuffed furniture. The distribution and abundance of dust mites is not uniform. Houses next door to each other of the same design can have vastly different mite populations. Nobody knows the exact numbers of mites in a given mattress or a carpet. Each mite would have to be removed and counted individually—an impossible task considering that the average mattress contains two million mites!

Dust mite populations fluctuate from season to season. In temperate climates, mite populations are highest in late summer and autumn and lowest in winter. The majority of dust mites love a warm, humid environment. This explains why dust mites thrive in damp rooms, especially in carpeted basements. Alterations in housing design have resulted in warmer, damper homes—a more favorable domestic microclimate for the dust mite. Mites die when the temperature falls below 50 degrees, or when humidity levels are kept at less than 50 percent. Due to the dry air at higher altitudes, house dust mite allergy is less common among people living in continental interiors or mountainous regions like Colorado than residents of sea-level maritime locales like Boston. A dormant or a dead mite is still an allergenic mite, as the mite's feces and body parts can trigger your allergy symptoms. The key symptoms that help to identify if you are mite-sensitive are sneezing and wheezing in the morning, or while vacuuming or making beds, and feeling better outside the home.

RISK FACTORS FOR ASTHMA

Innovative studies have shown that many asthma triggers are significant risk factors for people with allergic rhinitis and asthma. Let me explain what the term risk factor means. Allergists can accurately assess the severity of any hay fever season by counting the number of pollen grains in the air. We know that a prolonged period of dry, windy weather at the time of tree, grass, or ragweed pollination leads to high pollen counts that will trigger symptoms in millions of hay fever sufferers. Thus, a high pollen level is a "risk factor" for people with hay fever. Likewise, a high level of molds in the air is a risk if you are mold-allergic.

Cockroach Allergy

Cockroach allergy is a latecomer to the allergy scene, as its role in asthma was not recognized until 1967. The two most common cockroach species in the United States are the American and German cockroaches. The German cockroach is a small insect—approximately three-quarters of an inch in length—that infests kitchens and bathrooms. German cockroaches are important asthma triggers in older urban dwellings. You'll find the larger American cockroach in factories, schools, hospitals, and public buildings.

Seldom seen during the day, cockroaches are nocturnal creatures. Cockroach allergen, present in the saliva, feces, skin sheddings, and the dead bodies of the insect, are relatively large particles that only become airborne after a significant air disturbance. Thus, unlike animal allergic people, cockroach-sensitive individuals may not develop asthma immediately after entering a cockroach-infested home.

Cockroach activity has a seasonal pattern that usually peaks in the summer months. The National Cooperative Inner City Asthma Program found that children living in urban dwellings with cockroach infestation had more emergency room visits and hospitalizations for asthma. In this inner-city study, 85 percent of the homes surveyed had detectable levels of cockroach allergen.

Mold Aeroallergens

Molds or fungi are tiny plants lacking roots or stems that reproduce by releasing mold spores into the surrounding air. Indoor molds grow in damp, musty areas like cellars, garages, bathtubs, shower stalls, laundry rooms, and home humidifiers. Outdoor molds prefer the warm, moist, shady confines of mulch piles, black soil, gardens, and fallen leaves. Molds survive by digesting small amounts of decomposing foods or vegetable matter. A typical example of indoor mold is the fungus you see on stale bread or cheese. Mold that grows on aging foods is far less dangerous than the mold that grows in your bathroom, wet basement, or garden. Molds reproduce by releasing small spores into the air, creating airborne allergens similar to pollen. Mold-allergic people sneeze or wheeze after inhaling mold spores. There are tens of thousands of mold species, and only a few experts in the world are able to identify all of them. Under the microscope, mold spores look like golf balls without the logo.

Molds need four things to grow: food, air, proper temperatures, and water vapor. Molds thrive on garbage cans, houseplants, shower stalls, basement walls, and damp floors. Some molds reproduce when it rains, while others release their spores during the dry period that follows a rainy spell. Since molds eat just about anything and air is everywhere, the best way to inhibit mold growth is to control temperature and humidity.

In temperate climates, molds start to release their spores in early April or May. Outdoor mold levels usually peak in July or August. Mold symptoms may last until the first freeze or snowstorm. Molds are present year-round in the semitropical and tropical climates. The most intense exposure to molds in the United States occurs in the summer in the Midwest farm belts. When the ground freezes in early winter or it snows, outdoor molds cease to be a major problem. The most common asthma-inducing molds in North America are alternaria, penicillium, and cladosporium.

Mold Phobia

Mold mania or mold phobia is now the subject of intense controversy and litigation. Mold sleuths at the University of Arizona collected over 1,300 samples from 160 homes across the U.S. and found 100 percent of tested homes had mold infestation. The highest levels were found in Dallas, Texas, and New York State while the lowest levels were noted in Tampa, Florida. The highly publicized toxic mold, Stachybotrys, was found in only three of the 1,330 sampled homes. Not all mold symptoms are due to mold allergy. In one study of people who complained of mold symptoms, only 55 percent had positive skin tests to molds. Mold contamination is the result of tighter buildings and increased use of washing machines, vaporizers, and humidifiers. Molds produce a lot of toxins and VOCs (volatile organic compounds). Thus, many symptoms like headache and dizziness may be more of an irritant than an allergic reaction. Molds might be an important factor in the sick building syndrome. A Finland study found mold odors and visible mold caused more asthma in the workplace. Young Finnish women who smoked were more likely to have newly diagnosed asthma in these buildings.

Animal Allergens

A variety of domesticated animals live closely with humans, either as household companions, farm animals, or in research labs. It is estimated that over 100 million domestic animals reside in the United States, with dogs and cats being the most popular household pets. Tens of thousands of farmers and laboratory workers are exposed to animal allergens from cows, chickens, horses, pigs, rodents, rabbits, and guinea pigs. Animals raised for fur production like mink, fox, and raccoon are also recognized as occupational risks.

Dog Allergy

Dog ownership is common—there are approximately 50 million dogs in the United States. Studies have shown that approximately 35 percent of asthmatics are allergic to dogs. In a Los Alamos, New Mexico, survey 67 percent of asthmatic children were found to be allergic to dogs, and 62 percent were sensitized to cats. While dog allergen is found in homes and public places that do not house dogs, allergen levels are 250 times higher in homes where dogs reside. In homes that do house dogs, the highest allergen levels are found in carpets. The highest concentration in homes without a dog is found in upholstered living room furniture, suggesting that dog allergen is carried from home to home via the dog owner's clothing.

While there is some debate as to what part of the dog contains the most allergen, most allergen comes from skin scales and fur. Despite the claims of many dog breeders, there is no such thing as a non-allergenic dog or species. Even "hairless breeds" have significant amounts of allergen in their dander and skin. There is no evidence that longhaired dogs are more allergenic than shorthaired dogs.

There does seem to be a breed-to-breed or dog-to-dog difference. Some dogs or breeds just produce more allergen than others. One French investigator studied the allergen output from 141 dogs to determine if there were any differences between males and females, long- and shorthaired dogs, and castrated dogs. No significant differences in allergen levels were noted in these dogs. However, dogs who had dry skin or seborrhea had much higher levels of dog allergen, suggesting that aggressive skin care in dogs with skin problems may lower allergen output. In my own experience poodles, schnauzers, and some of the wire-haired terriers appear to be less allergenic than shorter-haired breeds like boxers, Dalmatians, and Labrador retrievers.

Cat Allergy

Cat allergy is a very common affliction. It is estimated that nearly 3 percent of the United States population, or 10 million Americans, are allergic to cats. According to a survey by the American Pet Product Manufacturers Association, approximately one in every three American homes now houses a cat or cats. That adds up to 28 million homes with an average of two cats per home, or roughly 60 million cats! Thanks to big strides in veterinary medicine, the average cat now has a lifespan of twenty or more years. It was once thought that the cat dander was the prime source of cat allergen. It is now known that the major sources of cat allergen are the proteins produced in the cat's saliva and sebaceous glands that attach to the cat's dander and hair.

Many people may not develop allergy or asthma symptoms for several years after a cat has been introduced into their home. The average exposure time needed to develop nasal allergies to cats is about two years, and for asthma it may be up to four to five years. The main in-home reservoirs of cat allergen are carpets, especially wall-to-wall carpeting, upholstered furniture, and bedding.

A French study found that male cats produce more allergen than female cats, and that the castration of males significantly lowers levels of cat allergen. These studies forewarned that castrated cats still produce enough allergen to affect most cat-allergic individuals. Like dog allergen, cat allergen is found everywhere, even in places where a cat has never resided, as cat allergen is carried from place to place on the owner's clothing.

Studies have shown that 50 percent of cat-allergic people have never owned a cat, attesting to the fact that cat allergen is a very powerful allergy and asthma trigger. Two of my five children and I are extremely sensitive to cats, yet we have never kept a cat in our home. Public buildings and the school setting are the most likely setting of cat allergen exposure.

In Chicago Children's Hospital Asthma Clinic, children with positive skin test to cats were three times more likely to have severe asthma.

All asthma caretakers know that the "asthma season" begins in the fall shortly after children return to school. In the past, the increase in the number of acute cases of asthma seen at this time of the year was attributed to weather changes, heating systems being turned on in the home, and viral respiratory infections. Swedish researchers may have found another reason why children start to wheeze when they go back to school. They studied ten children with mild asthma who were not exposed to animals in their own home. These animal-allergic children were symptom-free weeks before they returned to a school setting where there were significant concentrations of dog and cat allergen. One week after these children started school, analysis of secretions from their noses and lungs showed a dramatic increase in inflammatory or allergy blood cells. Thus, asymptomatic Swedish children with mild asthma had signs of airway inflammation one week after returning to classrooms infested with animal allergens, suggesting that exposure to animal allergens in the school is a major risk factor for asthma.

In a New Zealand study, where 62 percent of all students lived with a cat, investigators collected samples from school carpets and students' clothing. Large amounts of cat allergen were found on the students' clothing. Wool and polyester garments carried more cat allergen than cotton clothing, possibly due to more frequent laundering of cotton garments. Girls' clothing carried more cat allergen than boys' clothing, possibly because girls spend more time indoors. When cats were kept out of their bedrooms, students carried lower levels of cat allergen. High levels of cat allergen were found in school carpets where the children sat for several hours a day. These studies imply that sensitization to cat allergen is an evolving public health problem, in which exposure in the school setting may unknowingly sensitize susceptible children or trigger asthma attacks in people who do not keep cats in their own home. In my opinion this is a solid reason for new school construction or renovations to avoid carpeted surfaces in school classrooms.

Cat Asthma

There is an impressive number of new asthma patients who are allergic to cats. In many cases cat allergen is their major asthma trigger. I like to call this form of asthma "cat asthma."

A typical story of cat asthma is one where a cat is brought into the home, and on close questioning it becomes apparent that the patient began to have asthma symptoms a year or two after a cat was brought there, such as happens with a marriage. At first, most of these people will deny that the cat is bothering them, despite the fact they have a positive skin test to cat allergen. When I press the issue, they will admit that close contact with the cat will induce sneezing or itchy eyes. When I ask, "What happens when the cat licks you?" the answer is, "Oh, I get itchy and break out in welts." Upon further questioning, people with cat asthma will admit that their asthma worsens when they return home from school, work or vacations. They note substantial improvement when they leave home for any extended period of time.

Cat allergen, the most powerful of all antigens, is remarkably stable. It may remain in the environment long after a cat is removed from the home. Cats constantly lick their bodies and cover themselves with this potent allergen, which is then deposited throughout the home. Cat allergen, being the smallest of all inhaled allergens, penetrates very deep into the lung. I cannot overstate the importance of cat allergy and asthma. Some of my more dramatic "asthma cures" are the result of cats finally being removed from the home environment.

Preliminary data reveals that the number of cases of cat asthma has dramatically increased in the past decade. One recent survey estimated that cats now outnumber dogs 71 to 58 million. Thus, one of the reasons for the asthma epidemic may be due to the fact that there are more cats in more homes of individuals at risk for developing cat asthma.

The Pollen Allergens

Trees, grasses, weeds, and flowering plants all reproduce by producing pollen, the male sperm of the plant kingdom. Insects and wind currents transfer pollen from plant to plant. Pollens from trees, grasses, and weeds are light enough to be blown through the air and easily inhaled. The heavier pollens of flowering plants, like roses and privet hedges, that are carried about by low-flying insects, are much less allergenic than the wind-borne pollens.

Three major pollens affect hay fever sufferers and allergic asthmatics each calendar year, namely tree, grass, and weed pollens. In the southerly regions of the United States, tree pollination starts in February or March, while trees in the more northern areas of the United States do not pollinate until April or early May. Grass pollinates after the trees in late May or early June. The ragweed plant releases its pollen in late summer and early fall. The severity of any pollen season varies from year to year. The factors controlling pollination are air temperature and weather patterns. Cold, damp, rainy weather minimizes pollination, while hot, dry, windy weather accelerates it.

Ragweed Allergy

Some of the more potent hay fever and asthma-inducing pollen in the East and Midwest comes from the ragweed family. Members of the ragweed tribe include sunflower, cocklebur, goldenrod, and dandelion. Flowering plants like goldenrod and dandelion do not usually cause asthma or hay fever symptoms.

Ragweed starts to pollinate in mid-August, when the days become shorter and evening temperatures drop below 60 degrees. Thus, unlike the spring tree and summer grass pollination that starts in the south and proceeds in a northerly direction, ragweed pollination begins in the north and moves south. In most areas, ragweed pollination lasts for four to six weeks. Allergists used to think that ragweed victims only sneezed or wheezed when the plant was pollinating. People who continued to have symptoms in October and November were thought to be allergic to molds or house dust. Thanks to studies done at the Mayo Clinic, we now know that particles from dead ragweed plants remain in the air long after the plant stops pollinating and trigger sneezing and wheezing well past the first frost.

Latex Allergy

One particular form of allergy that has become much more common in the past decade is latex allergy. Latex is a natural product derived from the rubber tree, *Heavea brazilienis,* found in South America, Africa, and Southeast Asia. Latex is a common component of many medical supplies, including surgical gloves, stethoscopes, catheters, syringes, and tubing. It is used in thousands of consumer products, such as gloves, balloons, condoms, shoes, pacifiers, and rubber tires. Due to the increasing threat of infectious diseases, including AIDS and hepatitis B, the use of latex products has exploded, especially in the health-care industry. It is now estimated that between 10 and 15 percent of all health-care workers are sensitive to latex allergen.

Clinical symptoms of latex allergy may range from mild skin rash (hives or contact dermatitis) to sneezing, itchy eyes, asthma, or a full-blown, life-threatening anaphylactic reaction. Allergic and asthmatic individuals are more prone to developing latex allergy. Latex allergy sufferers also have a higher incidence of allergy to certain foods, in-cluding chestnuts, hazelnuts, and some tropical fruits, as these foods share common proteins with the latex allergen. Allergists used to think that individuals who sneezed or wheezed when they put on powdered latex gloves were allergic to the talc or powder that is released into the air when the gloves are put on or snapped off. We now know that the talcum powder carries the latex protein into the air. For this reason, many people who are latex-allergic have fewer symptoms when they use non-powdered gloves. In most cases, latex allergy develops after re-peated exposure.

Latex allergy can be diagnosed by the clinical history or by performing blood or skin tests. The only real treatment for latex allergy is avoidance of latex. Health-care providers, especially nurses, dentists, surgeons, and obstetricians, need to be aware of latex allergy, as any inadvertent exposure to latex during dental work, surgery, or labor and delivery has caused severe anaphylactic reactions, including many preventable, tragic fatalities. Hospitals and health-care facilities are now aware of the threat of latex allergy and provide latex-free environments for latex-allergic people.

CHAPTER SIX

The Dangers of Air Pollution and Asthma

Researchers have reexamined the role of air pollution in asthma. Atmospheric air pollutants come in several forms, including gases, aerosols, and small particles or particulate matter. Air pollutants vary in size from invisible, virus-sized molecules to easily seen, raindrop-sized particles. Outdoor air pollutants arise from factories, power plants, and the internal combustion engines of motorized cars, trucks, and buses. It is not surprising that outdoor and indoor air pollutants trigger asthma. An air pollutant inhaled into the lung can trigger an inflammatory response similar to that seen from inhaled aeroallergens.

The Ozone Ordeal

The four major outdoor air pollutants in our outdoor air are ozone, nitrogen dioxide, sulfur dioxide, and particulate matter. Ozone is the by-product of the interaction of sunlight and automobile exhaust fumes. Excess ozone creates smog, or the brown haze that permeates our atmosphere during the lazy, hazy days of summer. Ozone is a big problem for asthmatics in Los Angeles, California, where there is abundant sunlight and heavy automobile traffic. Ozone is a colorless gas with both good and bad qualities. The presence of ozone ten to thirty miles up in our stratosphere protects life on earth by screening out the sun's harmful ultraviolet rays and thereby minimizing dangers from the sun, including skin cancer. Ground-level ozone, on the other hand, is a direct irritant to the eyes, nose, throat, and lungs. Ozone production varies by season. The lowest concentrations occur during winter months, higher levels in spring, and peak levels in the summer. The ground-level ozone level that usually peaks in the late afternoon is directly proportional to atmospheric conditions and concentrations of exhaust emissions from motorized vehicles powered by fossil fuels.

Most asthmatics will tell you that they wheeze more during hot, humid weather. Studies show that high ozone levels lead to more hospitalizations and emergency room visits for asthma, and this risk is much greater in cigarette smokers. There is evidence that many people who are continuously exposed to high levels of ozone become increasingly tolerant to it. In one study, Los Angeles residents who were exposed to the highest levels of ozone in the United States tolerated more ozone exposure than visitors from Montreal, Canada, where ozone levels are much lower.

Several investigations have examined the effects of ozone on respiratory health in children. An increase in respiratory symptoms and a decline in lung function have been observed with high levels of ozone exposure. Children are more vulnerable to low levels of ozone exposure. The United States Environmental Protection Agency (EPA) data from Connecticut and Massachusetts found that children wheeze even when exposed to ozone levels that did not exceed EPA standards. A certain genetic make-up may predispose one to develop inflammation and lung scarring after ozone exposure. Ozone and other air pollutants may adversely affect individuals who carry this gene. Someday people with the "ozone gene" will be easily identified at an early age. Those who carry this gene could then be advised to live in areas or regions where ozone levels are low.

Nitrogen Dioxide

Nitrogen dioxide arises from the burning of fossil fuels in power plants and automobile exhaust emissions. Nitrogen dioxide levels are directly proportional to the number of cars, buses, and trucks on the road and, like ozone levels, peak during the late afternoon rush hour. Unlike ozone, nitrogen dioxide is also an important indoor air pollutant, as it is a by-product of cigarette smoke, gas stoves, and indoor kerosene heaters. Nitrogen dioxide levels are higher in homes with poorly ventilated gas cooking and heating appliances. Nitrogen dioxide also plays a role in public workplaces such as bus garages and ice-skating arenas. Several investigators have demonstrated that nitrogen dioxide levels are related to the frequency and duration of respiratory illness in children. This applies to outdoor as well as indoor exposure. Furthermore, people with allergic asthma have an increased response to inhaled allergens after a nitrogen dioxide exposure.

Sulfur Dioxide

Sulfur dioxide, a by-product of fossil fuel combustion in heavy industry, is more bothersome to people with asthma in cold, dry air versus warm, moist air. Sulfur dioxide gas is emitted into the air by coal-fired power plants, refineries, smelters, paper pulp mills, and food processing plants. The EPA considers sulfur dioxide a widespread outdoor air pollutant. People with asthma are especially sensitive to very low concentrations of sulfur dioxide—as little as one part per million. The combination of exposure to cold air and a high sulfur dioxide level has an additive effect.

Getting Particular about Particulates

Particulate matter is the term that refers to air particles arising from diesel or gasoline combustion, wood stoves, industrial smokestacks, and all other types of fuel combustion. Particulate matter is the most complex of all pollutants regulated by the EPA, which considers particulate matter to be one of the two major air pollutants—the other is ozone.

A high incidence of dust mite allergy has been found in neighborhoods with diesel air pollution. The level of diesel particles rises dramatically in the autumn, a time when asthma admissions also peak, suggesting that in some cities asthma admissions may be directly related to the level of diesel exhaust particles.

Epidemic Asthma

Several cities are hotspots for asthma epidemics. One of the first asthma epidemics occurred in the late 1920s and affected two hundred people in Toledo, Ohio, who lived within one mile of a mill which produced castor bean and linseed oil. Many people complained of asthma when the wind blew from the mill in their direction. Health investigators concluded that processing of castor beans produced a fine dust. Once the mill stopped processing castor beans, the asthma epidemic disappeared.

Another epidemic of asthma started in New Orleans in 1953 and lasted for fifteen years. Most of these asthma victims sought care at Charity Hospital. On one night in 1955, 350 people with asthma were treated in a twenty-four-hour period, two of whom died. In early November 1960, 200 people sought care in one day. Several theories for these episodes were studied, including exposure to fumes from a waste dump, aeroallergens associated with cold air masses moving into the city, and exposure to grain dust from barges moving down the Mississippi River. These New Orleans asthma outbreaks stopped suddenly in 1968 when the grain elevators along the river were modernized with new dust control equipment and filtering devices.

On Alert for Air Pollution

People with asthma who reside in areas subjected to thermal inversions, air pollution alerts, and asthma epidemics should monitor daily reports on weather and air pollution. Observe the following guidelines during air pollution alerts:

- Avoid unnecessary physical activity
- Avoid smoking and smoke-filled rooms
- Avoid dust and other irritants
- Avoid people with colds or the flu
- Stay indoors and use air conditioners
- Know your asthma medicines
- Exercise in the early morning, before pollution levels peak
- Run or cycle on less-congested roadways
- Travel or vacation in pollution-free areas
- Follow air pollution alerts via newspapers, radio, or TV
- Take additional medicine during air pollution alerts

Indoor Air Pollution

Thanks to the efforts of the EPA, we now know that indoor air pollution poses more of a public health problem than outdoor air pollution. Common indoor pollutants include microscopic-sized particles such as bacteria, yeast, house dust mites, molds, animal parts, pollens, and tobacco products. Air pollutants are also emitted from electrical appliances, hair dryers, and wood-, coal-, and gas-burning stoves and fireplaces. Additional sources include perfumes, colognes, household cleaners, deodorants, and hair sprays.

The EPA has found that air pollutants may be 100 times higher inside versus outside the home. Since Americans spend nearly 90 percent of their lives indoors, the threat of indoor air pollutants is now greater than outdoor air pollutants.

Parents Who Smoke

The risk for asthma posed by environmental tobacco smoke (ETS) is firmly established. Over the last fifteen years, there has been a steady accumulation of evidence that parents, especially mothers, who smoke in the home increase the risk of repeated respiratory infection and asthma in their children. A National Health Survey of 4,331 children found that if a mother smoked more than one-half pack of cigarettes per day, the risk of a child developing asthma was 2.6 times higher in the first year of life. Similar numbers came out of a study in Tucson, Arizona, where children of mothers who smoked more than ten cigarettes a day were 2.5 times more likely to develop asthma than children of nonsmoking mothers.

There is additional evidence that active cigarette smoking in adolescents and young adults also poses a risk for asthma. Common sense dictates that asthmatics should not smoke. Yet nearly one in every four asthmatics does smoke. Asthmatics who smoke do not respond as well to asthma medications. They greatly increase their chances of developing chronic bronchitis or crippling emphysema.

ETS exposure is potentially the most preventable risk factor for asthma. It is encouraging that the ban on smoking in public places in affluent countries has reduced exposure to ETS in the community. Unfortunately, the home is still the primary location for ETS exposure for children. Infants and children need to be protected from exposure to ETS in their own homes. Eliminating exposure to ETS reduces the incidence of serious respiratory infections in early childhood and may prevent asthma. It is essential that the medical community develop public-health strategies that focus on pregnant women and parents who smoke to prevent early ETS exposure in pregnant mothers and infants and children.

The Sick Building Syndrome

Modern-day construction methods employ energy-efficient building techniques to control fuel costs. Eighty-five percent of all new homes and buildings are energy efficient. People who live and work in these structures rarely breathe fresh outdoor air. In most newer office buildings, employees cannot open their office windows. This problem is not confined to new structures. Older apartment and office buildings are being remodeled with new energy-efficient conservation methods.

Heated or cooled air that is recycled through a closed system of air ducts may trigger a controversial set of symptoms called the sick building syndrome. Victims of the sick building syndrome experience headaches, frequent colds, sinus infections, nausea, eye irritation, skin rashes, and asthma.

Attack rates for asthma may approach 70 percent in some buildings. The sick building syndrome, also called building-related illness, is thought to be due to continuous inhalation of stale, recycled, contaminated air. Industry and governmental agencies have been slow to respond to the hazards posed by indoor air pollution. While Congress has appropriated millions of dollars for the study of air pollution, until recently less than 10 percent of air pollution expenditures was earmarked for indoor air studies. The National Institute of Occupational Safety and Health recommends that office ventilation systems provide outdoor air circulation at a minimum rate of twenty feet per minute per occupant in smoking areas, and five feet per minute in nonsmoking areas. There are no standards for home ventilation rates. If you suffer from "sick building syndrome," job relocation may be the only solution. One way to find out if you are living or working in a contaminated environment is to measure the level of carbon dioxide in the air. If the carbon dioxide level is high, it means that the heating or cooling system is not circulating enough fresh air. Building managers often shut down the fresh air intake to control heating or cooling costs. Simply increasing the intake of fresh air into the system will solve a lot of problems when office windows cannot be opened.

Hot Air Heating Systems
The typical forced-hot-air heating system in a home or office building recycles air through vents after it has been warmed or cooled by an oil- or gas-fired furnace or heat exchanger. Low costs entice builders and developers to install hot air systems in new homes, apartments, and condominiums. Hot air systems pose a serious threat to asthmatics, as

their vents constantly recycle dust, mold, pollen, bacteria, and animal parts throughout the dwelling.

The allergic asthmatic living in a home heated by forced hot air must take some special precautions. The system should be properly filtered and maintained. Avoid using central humidifiers that tend to become infested with molds. Family room and bedroom air vents should be covered with cheesecloth or fiberglass filters. In some cases it may be necessary to seal off the ducts and install supplemental electric heat. Hot air systems should be vacuumed or professionally cleaned before the start of each heating season. Sometimes, I find it necessary to advise a sick asthmatic to move out of a rented home or apartment with hot air heat. Tenants who feel they are at the mercy of a tight lease or rental agreement usually have no problem breaking their lease after I write a letter to their landlord stating that their present environment poses a significant health hazard.

Wood and Coal Stoves

The ancient fossil fuels, wood and coal, are man's oldest source of energy. Wood and coal combustion produces more toxins and air pollutants than oil or gas combustion. In communities where wood stoves are used, wintertime air inversions trap wood smoke and produce a ground-hugging layer of contaminated outdoor air pollutants, particles, and toxins that aggravate asthma. A typical wood stove produces up to eighty pounds of unburned material per cord of wood. Each day a wood stove emits as much carbon monoxide as an automobile does on a fifty-mile trip.

There is no question that wood and coal stoves can aggravate asthma, but convincing stove owners is another matter. Families who save hundreds of dollars a year in heating costs are understandably reluctant to give up their stoves. I usually recommend turning the stove off for three to four weeks on a trial basis. If asthma improves while the stove is off, or recurs when the stove is turned back on, the stove should be permanently shut down.

Controlling Indoor Air Pollution

How does one address air quality within your own home? Dr. Rebecca Bascom, Chief of Pulmonary Medicine at Penn State University, has outlined a five-step, walk-through approach to evaluate the major areas in your home.

Step 1. Look at the overall structure of the home. The home may be too tightly insulated, preventing the exchange of fresh air. While such a home has lower heating and cooling costs, indoor air pollutants are easily trapped. Make sure combustible appliances like gas stoves, furnaces, and hot water heaters are professionally installed and vented to the outdoors. If you are building a new home or remodeling your kitchen, consider installing an electric stove.

Step 2. Look at things inside your home. New rugs, furniture, or flooring may emit gas or chemicals months after they are installed. Many European countries do not allow occupants of new buildings to enter the structure for several months after construction has been completed.

Step 3. Evaluate activities in the home. Eliminate indoor smoking. Minimize use of aerosol and spray can products. Avoid personal products with strong odors or scents. Avoid using pesticides within the home.

Step 4. Evaluate how air moves in and around your home. Dr. Bascom quotes an old adage, "The solution to pollution is dilution." A regular supply of fresh air is essential for good indoor air quality. Houses heated or cooled with central air systems are of particular concern. Make sure that air-conditioning systems are checked and are free of excess condensation and molds. Filters should be changed on a regular basis. Hot air heating ducts should be professionally vacuumed and cleaned annually. Poor maintenance of these systems encourages the build-up of dust particles, mold, and bacteria.

Step 5. Determine how water and humidity move in and around your home. Water vapor in the air produces what is known as humidity. Humidity levels above 50 percent provide an ideal growth environment for dust mites, molds, and bacteria. Control indoor humidity levels, especially in damp basements, with properly functioning air conditioners or home dehumidifiers. Condensation on heating or air-conditioning ducts is usually a sign of excess humidity. Insulation of these ducts may be necessary. An instrument called a hygrometer, sold in home improvement outlets or hardware stores, can measure indoor humidity levels.

Warm Days, Cool Nights, and Thunderstorms

Many asthma relapses and admissions commonly occur in the months characterized by warmer days and colder nights, especially on days characterized by a mid-afternoon temperature of 60 or so degrees Fahrenheit. In the late afternoon or early evening, these comfortable daytime temperatures rapidly plunge down to the low forties or high thirties. I believe this rapid and wide swing in outdoor temperature is a risk factor for some people with asthma. Many asthma sufferers and parents of asthmatic children say that asthma is much worse on the days when this late afternoon-early evening temperature change is most extreme. Savvy emergency room nurses know that these are the evenings, especially Halloween night, when the emergency room will be busy treating wheezy or croupy trick-or-treaters.

Mini-asthma epidemics have been linked to thunderstorm activity in England and Europe. In 1997, British doctors tracked phone calls made after thunderstorms and found a tenfold increase in calls to doctors for asthma care immediately after a thunderstorm. Asthmatics affected by thunderstorms should go indoors, stay in air-conditioned automobiles, or take their preventative asthma medicines when such storms are approaching their areas, especially during the pollen seasons.

CHAPTER SEVEN

Food Allergy and Asthma

Foodstuffs, beverages, and chemical additives can trigger asthma and allergic reactions. The average human being consumes five to six thousand pounds of foodstuffs and chemical additives and several thousand gallons of beverages over a 70- to 80-year life span. Normally our intestinal tract and digestive system are incredibly efficient organs that separate the helpful from harmful foods and beverages. However, in a small percentage of individuals, ingested foods and beverages trigger an allergic reaction. While more than two hundred foodstuffs can cause an allergic reaction, most reactions are caused by the "big eight": peanuts, tree nuts, fish, shellfish, milk, eggs, wheat, and soybeans.

A recent survey found that between one and two percent of adults are allergic to peanuts or tree nuts, and another two percent of adults are allergic to other foods, especially fish and shellfish. These numbers add up to about 7 million Americans having food allergies. The incidence of food allergy is highest in infancy and early childhood, presumably due to the immaturity of the gastrointestinal tract's immune system. Six to eight percent of children under age four have one or more food allergies. Most children will outgrow their food allergy by age ten, when the prevalence of food allergy approaches adult levels.

Children with eczema, who have a much higher incidence of food allergy, are more likely to be allergic to milk, eggs, peanuts, or tree nuts. Five percent of children with asthma have food allergies, and about one percent are prone to a severe food reaction.

Nearly one in every four American families has altered their dietary habits because of the perception that one or more members of their family suffer from a food allergy. While some surveys imply that 25 percent of the population has a food allergy or an adverse food reaction, only one in every ten food reactions is a true immunological reaction driven by the allergic or IgE antibody response.

Killed by a Kiss

The diagnosis of food allergy requires a careful medical history followed up by allergy skin or blood tests. Unfortunately, there is a wide discrepancy between the perceptions of patients and physicians regarding food allergy. Food allergy is often erroneously blamed for a variety of conditions, including asthma. When food does induce asthma, the most common inciting foods are peanuts, tree nuts, and shellfish. The time between food ingestion and the onset of wheezing is usually quite brief—minutes to hours. In the majority of cases, the amount of food required to induce symptoms is quite small. Sometimes, merely inhaling odors from a cooking food or being exposed to airborne food particles will cause wheezing or an allergic reaction.

In her excellent book *The Allergy Bible* (Readers Digest Publications, 2001), Linda Gamlin describes how food-allergic people can be killed by a kiss. Gamlin depicts a young man with fish allergy who required emergency care after being kissed by his girlfriend who had just eaten mackerel. In another case, a peanut-allergic child experienced a severe allergic reaction after he was kissed by his aunt who had just eaten some peanuts.

When foods do trigger wheezing, people often experience other allergic symptoms, such as swelling or edema, hives, shock, and even complete cardiovascular collapse. When hives are the only symptom, the food reaction is usually mild. When lung, heart, and blood vessels are involved, or if the throat closes up, the allergic reaction becomes a severe, life-threatening medical emergency called anaphylaxis. When the clinical history reveals a severe, life-threatening or anaphylactic reaction, skin testing may be dangerous, as it could trigger an acute allergic reaction. Blood or RAST testing is the preferred method for detecting the offending food in such cases. Skin testing to foods is not as accurate as skin testing to airborne allergens. A positive skin test to a food does not always indicate the presence of food allergy, as studies have shown that only 40 percent of people with a positive skin test react to a food challenge.

Most children who are allergic to eggs, cow's milk, soy, and wheat eventually outgrow these food allergies by age three or four. Unfortunately, allergy to peanuts, tree nuts, or shellfish is not always outgrown. A recent study in England found that only 20 percent of school-aged children who had a peanut reaction in infancy became tolerant to the food later on in childhood. Those children who did outgrow their peanut allergy had smaller skin test reactions to peanuts, and were less likely to have eczema or asthma.

Skin tests are one way to determine if a child has outgrown a food allergy. A negative test is a good indicator that a food allergy has resolved. Sometimes, a food allergy skin test remains positive long after the food allergy is outgrown. This is called a false positive skin test. In these cases a careful food challenge may be the only way to determine the presence or absence of a food allergy. Sometimes, food allergies begin in adulthood, especially fruit and vegetable allergy. Most allergic reactions to fresh fruits and vegetables are mild and not life-threatening events. People with fruit and vegetable allergy often have significant tree pollen allergy.

Food Anaphylaxis—Yet Another Epidemic

Food allergy can trigger severe, life-threatening reactions, or anaphylaxis, especially in people who are allergic to peanuts or tree nuts. It is estimated that two hundred people die per year in the United States from fatal food reactions. Four independent studies from the United States and England looked at emergency room records to determine the cause of severe allergic reactions that required an emergency room visit. The leading cause by far for this type of emergency visit was a food allergy, which accounted for one in every three visits. Food allergy has not been spared by the asthma-allergy epidemic. There is a growing concern about the rising incidence of severe allergic reactions to foods, which has paralleled the rise in asthma and other allergic diseases. The type of allergic reaction that is generating the most concern is life-threatening anaphylaxis.

Staying Alert for Anaphylaxis

The most common causes for anaphylactic reactions are foods, aspirin-like drugs, antibiotics, latex, and stinging insects. Anaphylaxis is more frequent and more severe in adults, especially women. Severe food reactions are more likely to occur in atopic or allergic people who are better allergic antibody or IgE producers. Anaphylaxis can strike the skin, gastrointestinal tract, and respiratory and cardiovascular systems. Skin symptoms of anaphylaxis are facial flushing, itchiness, excess sweating, hives (urticaria), and swelling (angioedema). Gastrointestinal symptoms include nausea, vomiting, abdominal cramps, and diarrhea. In severe cases cardiorespiratory symptoms cause dizziness, low blood pressure (fainting or collapse), swelling in the throat, shortness of breath, coughing, and wheezing. Not all these symptoms have to be present, nor do they appear in any special order. In most cases anaphylaxis symptoms begin within minutes or one to two hours after exposure to the offending allergen. Sometimes, the reaction may be delayed for several hours.

One dangerous type of anaphylaxis is called biphasic anaphylaxis, where the victim has an immediate reaction that resolves with appropriate treatment and then recurs several hours later. The biggest danger of biphasic anaphylaxis is that people may respond promptly to their initial emergency room treatment and be prematurely discharged, only to experience a second or biphasic reaction several hours after they have left the emergency room. The take-home message here for emergency room docs and nurses is that anyone who experiences a moderate to severe anaphylactic reaction, especially if they have low blood pressure, should be observed in the emergency room for six to eight hours before being sent home.

Treatment of Anaphylaxis

The treatment of choice in anaphylaxis is epinephrine or adrenaline, the hormone produced by our adrenal gland. There are few major risks to epinephrine.

Epinephrine increases heart rate and blood pressure, constricts blood vessels, and opens up narrowed airways. Minor side effects include a pounding heart, pallor, dizziness, tremors, and headache. In the clinic or hospital setting, epinephrine is given by injection. Automatic epinephrine injector kits are available for use in the home, at school, or in public places. The best kit is the EpiPen, which is easy to use and carry. The safest and most effective place to inject the EpiPen is the outer thigh muscle.

Anyone who experiences symptoms of an allergic or anaphylactic reaction should take Benadryl, an antihistamine; self-administer the EpiPen; and immediately proceed to the nearest hospital. You should carry extra epinephrine on trips or while camping, boating, golfing, or engaging in activities where immediate medical care is not readily available. Recent studies on compliance in people who are food allergic are discouraging. Only 20 percent of people advised to carry an EpiPen had it with them when they experienced a reaction to a known antigen. Sadly, many of these reactions resulted in death, especially in asthmatics. The take-home message here is clear! Carry your EpiPen at all times—it may save your life.

For further information on anaphylaxis, I suggest you contact Media Works in Canada. Media Works has produced an excellent video and booklet for anaphylactic victims and their families. Kimberly Curran, a video producer and mother of a child with severe peanut allergy, initiated this work. These materials are sponsored by the Anaphylaxis Foundation of Canada and endorsed by the Canadian Society of Allergy and Clinical Immunology. Contact Media Works @ 141 Stuart Street, Cobourg, Ontario, Canada K9A 2Y1. Phone 905-373-9324 or www.mediaworkstudio.tripod.com

A New Threat—Asthma and Food Anaphylaxis

The frequency of severe, life-threatening and fatal reactions to foods in people with asthma has risen dramatically over the past two decades. Tragically, the majority of these fatalities occur in children and young adults with asthma who were fully aware of their preexisting food allergy. Case studies have found that most near-fatal or fatal anaphylactic reactions due to foods occur in asthmatics who are severely allergic to peanuts, tree nuts, or shellfish. After accidental ingestion of the offending foods, these unfortunate individuals did not take or were not given the proper emergency care that could have saved their lives. Such care includes prompt administration of epinephrine (EpiPen) and Benadryl, and immediate transport to an emergency facility.

Thirty-two cases of fatal food reactions were reviewed in the *Journal of Allergy and Clinical Immunology* in January 2001. Most of these people were adolescents or young adults. Only three of them were less than ten years of age. All but one had asthma, 90 percent of deaths were due to peanut or tree nut ingestion, and all but one of these people were aware of a preexisting peanut or tree nut allergy. The two deaths to fish and milk ingestion occurred in younger children. Only three people had their EpiPen available. The following two cases typify fatal food anaphylaxis:

Case 1. BF was a nine-year-old male with asthma and nut allergy who was given some peanut candy by a classmate in school. Ninety minutes later he went to the nurse's office complaining of abdominal pain. Unfortunately, the school nurse was not aware of his peanut allergy. Within twenty minutes he began to vomit and have difficulty breathing and three hours after ingesting the peanut-laced candy he died in a local emergency room.

Clearly this was a preventable death, which points out the need for education of all caretakers of children as well as the need to administer epinephrine immediately after the signs and symptoms of a food reaction begin, even if the symptoms are mild in nature.

Case 2. AF was a 32-year-old female with chronic asthma and a history of peanut and nut allergy since childhood. Her asthma was considered to be moderate in severity as she experienced four to five relapses per year that required prednisone. She had no prior history of emergency room visits or hospitalizations for asthma. In June 1990, while driving and eating a Danish that contained a hidden nut, she began to wheeze and she drove herself to a local emergency room where she was treated with epinephrine, Benadryl, and Solumedrol (a cortisone drug). She improved rapidly and was discharged in about two hours. This proved to be a mistake. On the way home, her asthma recurred. She drove back to the emergency room, collapsed in the parking lot, and was found in acute respiratory arrest. She was immediately admitted to an intensive care unit, placed on a respirator, and subsequently recovered. Over the next four years, her asthma was relatively stable. In January 1994, while dining at a mall restaurant, she ordered a dish with pesto sauce, which according to her waiter did not contain any nuts. Tragically, the pesto sauce contained hidden walnuts and she immediately experienced a severe anaphylactic reaction and arrived in the local emergency room in a comatose state and died several days later.

The take-home message of this heartbreaking case is that waiters don't prepare your food. If you are food-allergic, speak with the restaurant manager or even the chef before ordering foods that may contain hidden food allergens. People must be taught to read menus and food labels and to be very vigilant in restaurants where cross-contamination or spatula carryover may occur.

Exercise-Induced Anaphylaxis

One unique form of anaphylaxis is called exercise-induced anaphylaxis. In 1980, Doctors Albert Sheffer and Frank Austin, researchers from Harvard University, described a group of adolescents and young adults who during or shortly after exercise felt warm and itchy, developed hives or swelling, or experienced cardiovascular collapse. Additional symptoms included wheezing and stomach cramps. This reaction was more likely to occur in young athletes during vigorous exercise in warmer weather. Sheffer and Austin labeled this syndrome exercise-induced anaphylaxis.

In 1983, Doctor Jordan Fink from the University of Wisconsin reported additional cases of young athletes with exercise-induced anaphylaxis. Fink's patients related that they only experienced symptoms when they ate certain foods prior to exercising. The most common foods that predisposed them to exercise-induced anaphylaxis were celery and carrots. Many subsequent reports have described other foods, including fish, nuts, and wheat, capable of triggering exercise-induced anaphylaxis. It is postulated that people with food-related, exercise-induced anaphylaxis have a subtle or unrecognized allergy to certain foods that only manifests itself when the offending food allergen is rapidly absorbed during or after exercise. The treatment of exercise-induced anaphylaxis is quite basic. First, if it is food-related, one must avoid the triggering food before exercising. It may also be helpful to avoid exercising in warmer weather. Allergy skin tests, especially with fresh foods, often help identify the offending food. Victims of exercise-induced anaphylaxis should not exercise alone, and should always carry an emergency, self-injectable epinephrine kit.

Oral Allergy Syndrome

Allergy specialists have long been aware that many hay fever sufferers complain of an itchy mouth, tongue, or lips after eating fresh fruits and vegetables, like apples, pears, peaches, celery, carrots, and members of the melon family. Yet they have no problems with cooked foods, such as apple pie, canned fruits, or heated vegetables. Any given food may contain ten to thirty proteins, of which only a few act as an allergen. Heating or cooking a food often denatures the allergenic food protein. Some food allergens have a striking resemblance to pollen and latex allergens. This observation explains why some pollen- and latex-sensitive individuals experience an itchy mouth or throat when they eat these fruits and vegetables, especially in their raw state. For example, people with tree pollen allergy may have difficulty eating raw apples, pears, peaches, carrots, or celery.

Ragweed-sensitive individuals experience symptoms after eating melons or bananas. Latex-allergic patients may react to chestnuts, bananas, avocado, and kiwi fruit. This cross-reactivity is due to a shared enzyme that protects plants and fruits against insects. Latex comes from the sap of the rubber tree, and the tree is laced with this enzyme to protect it from insects. This syndrome has been labeled the Oral Allergy Syndrome. Fortunately, it is usually a mild reaction localized to the mouth or tongue. Treatment is simple—avoid the offending food, especially in its raw or uncooked state.

Treatment of Food Allergy

Once a specific food has been identified as an asthma or allergy trigger, the treatment is avoidance. People with asthma and food allergy should be aware that most foods belong to a food group or a food family. An allergy to one member of a specific food family often means that ingestion of other members of the same food family will cause an allergic reaction. For example, if you are allergic to lobster, a member of the crustacean family, you are quite likely to experience an allergic reaction when you eat other crustaceans like crab or shrimp. Can the lobster-sensitive person eat fried clams or scallops? The answer is usually yes.

Unfortunately, many doctors have forgotten their basic biology. When confronted with a patient with a crustacean allergy, they recommend avoiding all forms of shellfish or seafood. This is unnecessary, as shellfish like clams, oysters, and scallops belong to the mollusk family, and do not usually cross-react with crustaceans. In other words, the patient with lobster allergy may not be allergic to clams, oysters, or scallops. Properly performed skin or RAST tests may help sort out food allergies. Food-sensitive asthmatics should not experiment with food groups without the approval of their doctor or allergy specialist. They should also consult their physician, nutrition center, or local library for a complete list of foods and food families.

People with peanut allergy often ask if they can eat other nuts, like walnuts or pecans. Likewise, patients with tree nut allergy want to know if they can safely ingest peanuts or peanut butter. Believe it or not, peanuts are not true nuts. They are members of the legume vegetable family that includes peas, soybeans, and beans. On the other hand, true nuts such as walnuts, almonds, and pecans belong to the tree nut family. Dr. Hugh Sampson has helped answer these questions. He conducted an extensive survey of children with peanut and tree nut allergy and found that one in every three peanut-allergic patients were sensitive to tree nuts. The bottom line is that one can never predict when the peanut-allergic patient will become tree-nut-allergic and vice versa.

Thus, it is best for a peanut-sensitive or tree-nut-sensitive person to avoid all forms of peanuts and tree nuts. Sampson's survey also found that 30 percent of people who are tree-nut-allergic experienced an accidental ingestion of tree nuts, and more than half of peanut-allergic children had two or more accidental encounters with peanuts within five years of their first peanut reaction. The modes of accidental ingestion included hidden ingredients in processed foods, cross-contamination of foods, sharing food with friends, skin contact with peanut butter in classroom and day care centers, and hidden foods in restaurants, especially Asian restaurants.

People with asthma and peanut or tree nut allergy should avoid most if not all packaged foods. An unpublished FDA study found that only half of 85 candy, ice cream, and baked-good food plants in Wisconsin and Minnesota were checking to see if the ingredients on their labels matched the ingredients in the foods. Half of these FDA-surveyed plants were turning out foods that contained allergens not listed on their label. Many factories used the same utensils that were supposed to be used in allergen-free foods when making foods with peanuts or eggs. One in every four FDA-sampled foods contained undisclosed peanut allergen. Several important points to remember in preventing food allergy include:

- Educate younger siblings, babysitters, nannies, and grandparents.
- Keep epinephrine (EpiPen) kits available everywhere, especially in remote locales—golfing, boating, and hiking.
- Maintain a peanut- and tree-nut-free home.
- Take special precautions in day care and school settings, including separate eating tables, no food swapping or trading eating utensils, and the washing of hands, tables, and toys after eating.
- Encourage teachers and school nurses to develop an action plan for food-allergic children. Families and health-care providers must partner with parents, staff, and school nurses in food-allergy education.
- Allow responsible students to carry their own EpiPen.
- Do not discriminate or isolate these students, as they are fully protected by federal disability laws.

The Food Allergy and Anaphylaxis Network

I strongly urge any patient or family affected by food allergies to join the Food Allergy and Anaphylaxis Network or FAAN. This excellent, proactive national organization provides support and educational materials for food allergy sufferers and their families. FAAN's many publications include allergen-free recipes, timely alerts when processed foods become contaminated with food allergens, booklets, videos, and a well-thought-out School Allergy Program. FAAN also publishes a bimonthly newsletter for its members. *Food Allergy News for Physicians* is distributed to ten thousand pediatricians throughout the country. FAAN has an e-newsletter for teens called *Food Allergy News for Teens*. You can sign up for this newsletter through FAAN's Web site. FAAN is also working closely with the Federal Aviation Administration and lobbying for placement of self-injectors of epinephrine in commercial aircraft emergency medical kits. They are also encouraging Emergency Medical Services to allow all EMTs to administer epinephrine. For additional information contact FAAN at 10400 Eaton Place, Suite 107, Fairfax, VA 22030-2208. Telephone: 1-800-929-4040 or 703-691-3179. Fax: 703-691-2713. www.foodallergy.org

The Peanut Allergy Answer Book

My good friend and colleague, Dr. Michael Young, has written a very informative resource book for parents of children afflicted with peanut and tree nut allergy—*The Peanut Allergy Answer Book* (Fair Winds Press, 2001). The easy-to-read, question-and-answer format helps relieve the anxiety and frustration often associated with food allergy and anaphylaxis. Young's collection of illustrative cases helps to explain the up-to-date scientific information for those who want to learn more about peanut allergy. I highly recommend this book to all my patients, parents, caregivers, and health-care providers who deal with peanut or tree nut allergy.

Sulfite-Induced Asthma

If you read the labels on foods and beverages you purchase in your local supermarket, you are fully aware that thousands of agents are added to the foodstuffs we consume on a daily basis. Such additives include preservatives, stabilizers, conditioners, thickeners, colorings, and flavorings. It is somewhat amazing that despite the widespread use of food additives, relatively few of these chemicals trigger asthma or other allergic reactions. One of the few additives that may trigger asthma is the sulfite chemical called metabisulfite. Sulfites have been used for centuries to preserve raw potatoes, seafood, and fresh vegetables. The Romans were the first to discover that sulfites prevented wine from turning into vinegar. Ingestion of large amounts of sulfites by normal individuals is usually quite safe. Not so for those susceptible asthmatics in whom sulfites may trigger severe asthma attacks. Sulfite sensitivity is rare in children, and mainly occurs in adults with persistent asthma.

From 1980 to 1998 the FDA received over one thousand reports of severe sulfite reactions, of which twelve were fatal episodes. More than 90 percent of these sulfite reactions occurred away from home, in restaurants. The FDA and National Restaurant Association responded to the threat of sulfite sensitivity by developing training programs and handouts for food manufacturers, restaurant personnel, and consumers. After the FDA prohibited sulfite use in restaurants and supermarkets and required labeling disclosure when the sulfite concentration exceeded ten parts per million, the incidence of sulfite reactions dropped dramatically—to about ten a year. It appears that restaurant chefs were using too much sulfite on salad bar fruits and vegetables.

The exact incidence of sulfite-sensitive asthma is unknown. Drs. Donald Stevenson and Ronald Simon, of La Jolla, California, estimate that five to ten percent of all adult asthmatics may be sulfite sensitive. If their figures are correct, there may be five hundred thousand sulfite-sensitive asthmatics in the United States. At first I doubted these estimates and thought sulfite asthma was a rare problem. But now that I am looking for it, I find so-called "Restaurant-Induced Asthma" is not all that uncommon. Fresh shrimp and some factory-prepared foods, like mashed potato flakes or fried potatoes, still contain sulfites, as do most beers and imported wines. If you can drink beer or wine, you are not sulfite sensitive, as most domestic and imported beers and wines contain sulfites. It is really up to the consumer to be aware of the potential sources of sulfites. (See Table 7.1.)

Several other food additives and colorings have the reputation of inducing asthma, including tartrazine or FD&C Yellow Dye Number 5. This dye, a derivative of coal tar, is commonly used to color foods, like margarine, yellow. Tartrazine is widely avoided by many people with asthma. This is unnecessary, as the threat of tartrazine allergy is grossly overrated. Similar concerns have been raised about other food additives and chemicals, including sodium benzoate, BHA, and BHT. Tests in large asthmatic populations have failed to implicate these chemical additives as important asthma triggers.

MSG-Induced Asthma

Individuals with MSG, or monosodium glutamate, sensitivity usually experience facial flushing and a generalized tingling sensation after consuming MSG. Since Chinese foods frequently contain large amounts of MSG, this condition is commonly known as the "Chinese

TABLE 7.1
FOODS AND BEVERAGES THAT CONTAIN SULFITES

• Wine, beer, and cider	• Avocados
• Fruit drinks	• Corn sweeteners
• Fresh shrimp	• Salad bars
• Potatoes, French fries	• Dried fruits, grapes
• Beet sugar	• Baked goods

Restaurant Syndrome." In the early 1980s a possible association between MSG and asthma was raised, as several studies described patients who developed asthma-like symptoms after ingesting Chinese food. Since MSG is a widely used dietary supplement (we normally ingest one gram of MSG per day) the possibility that MSG might play a major role in asthma was raised.

In 1999, doctors from the Scripps Research Institute in La Jolla, California, carefully challenged 100 asthmatics with MSG, and none of these people developed asthma symptoms or had any change in their lung functions. Many people who thought they were sensitive to MSG were found to have gastroesophageal reflux disease, or anxiety or depression that caused them to overstate their fear of MSG products. Dr. Raif Geha of Harvard University challenged 130 people who thought they were sensitive to MSG with a large test dose of MSG and found only a low level of MSG sensitivity. On the basis of these two studies and my own professional experience, I do not consider MSG to be an important asthma trigger.

Alcohol-Induced Asthma

In contrast to MSG, many of my patients with asthma tell me that ingestion of beer, wine, or grain alcohol frequently triggers sneezing, nasal congestion, or wheezing. Wine, especially red wine, is a more frequent offender than beer or grain alcohol. In a survey in Western Australia, one in every three asthmatics noted that alcoholic drinks worsened their asthma. Wines were the most frequent offenders, with a response time of less than one hour. Wine-induced asthma that was mild to moderate in severity was more common in women. I used to think that alcohol-induced asthma was due to the sulfite preservatives added to alcoholic beverages to prevent spoilage, but it was always a puzzle why not all alcoholic beverages triggered asthma.

It appears Japanese investigators have come up with the answer. Alcohol-induced asthma in Japan has been well documented, as more than half of asthmatic people in Japan wheeze after consuming alcohol. Studies found that many Japanese people have a genetically determined enzyme defect that prevents the breakdown of acetaldehyde, a by-product of alcohol. High levels of acetaldehyde apparently trigger the release of histamine from mast cells, which leads to bronchospasm and wheezing. Japanese researchers have published a small study on thirteen patients that provides some hope for asthmatics who enjoy drinking beer or wine, as pretreatment with antihistamines could block alcohol-induced asthma.

Facts and Findings

Right now the only effective treatment for food or chemical-induced allergy or asthma is avoidance and education. When indicated, the treatment of choice is an inhaled asthma rescue drug, an antihistamine, and immediate use of epinephrine and prompt transport to a local emergency room. Biotech research in food allergy is focusing on ways to prevent food allergy, including anti-IgE therapy and allergy injections with highly purified, less allergenic proteins. Doctors from Denver's NJH (National Jewish Hospital) have published the preliminary results of treatment with an experimental drug (TNX-901) for peanut allergy. A total of eighty-four NJH patients with peanut allergy received either TNX-901 or a placebo for four weeks. The treated group was able to tolerate an average of nine peanuts after treatment. Research studies like these will eventually lead to a "prevention or cure" for food allergy.

Another new piece of animal research may also be important. Australians found that mice who were fed antacids were more likely to develop allergic antibodies to foods, implying that antacids may lower the acid content of the stomach and leave food proteins more intact and more likely to trigger antibody formation. Thus, the possibility that infants treated for GERD or gastroesophageal reflux disease with acid-lowering drugs may be more likely to develop a food allergy at a young age needs to be studied.

CHAPTER EIGHT

Infections and Asthma

Viral Infections

There is no doubt that the most important asthma trigger other than an aeroallergen is a viral infection or the common cold. More than 240 viruses are capable of causing a common cold. A virus is a living biologic particle that has the ability to invade a specific cell and use the metabolic machinery of the invaded cell to duplicate itself. Viruses are actually parasites. They cannot survive on their own, but must live off the chemicals of the invaded cell. All viruses are composed of a core surrounded by a protein shell. Every virus has the ability to enter a host cell, duplicate itself, and form more viral particles that are then released into the surrounding tissue. Once inside a cell, a virus uses the cell's enzymes and metabolic machinery to reproduce proteins and building blocks required to duplicate itself. The final stage in the life cycle of a virus depends on its ability to be transmitted from one victim to another.

Viruses that cause respiratory symptoms are transmitted through touching, coughing, or sneezing. Infected secretions from infected individuals contain various-sized droplets. Larger droplets settle on handkerchiefs, hands, and other surfaces. Smaller droplets remain airborne and are inhaled into the nose and lower airways, where they cause infection.

Viral Infections in Childhood

One study found that four out of every ten hospitalizations for childhood asthma were caused by a common cold virus. Different viruses strike different age groups. Infants and children are more susceptible to the RSV virus and mycoplasma infections. Rhinovirus may be the most important cause of infection-induced asthma in older children. Adult asthmatics are more likely to be infected with the influenza or rhinoviruses. There are clues as to why people with allergies and asthma are prone to repeated colds and asthma relapses. Some allergic individuals are more likely to produce an allergic or IgE antibody to certain viruses. Doctors also know that the common cold is more likely to be transmitted by hand-to-mouth contact than by droplets produced by coughing or sneezing. Upper respiratory tract viruses cause nasal congestion, which leads to long periods of mouth breathing. Air breathed through the mouth is not subject to the warming and humidifying that occurs in the nose, and may trigger bronchospasm in the same way that cold and dry air precipitates exercise-induced asthma.

Wheezing in children has traditionally been divided into two classes: wheezy bronchitis precipitated by a viral infection, and classic asthma. Epidemiological studies that looked at asthma attacks provide evidence for virus involvement. One eleven-year-long study done in London, England, found there was no association between admission rates and changes in weather or aeroallergen exposure. Asthma admissions coincided with the beginning of school terms when children were exposed to viruses in their classrooms. Respiratory viruses were associated with one in every four episodes of wheezing in these London schoolchildren. British asthma doctors have labeled the third Monday in September as "Black Monday." After the start of the school year, the number of hospital admissions throughout Britain can increase from an average of twenty to thirty per day up to three hundred on the third Monday in September. It is thought that the return to school and close exposure to other classmates with viral infections sets off this asthma outbreak.

A prospective study of thirty-two young children admitted to the National Jewish Hospital found that one-third of wheezy episodes in the first year of life were associated with a viral infection. The most common asthma-triggering virus was RSV.

RSV Infection

RSV or respiratory syncytial virus is a viral infection of infants and young children that triggers nearly one hundred thousand hospitalizations a year, costing $300 million. RSV illness is often called bronchiolitis. In older children and adults, bronchiolitis may be a milder disease, often presenting as a simple cold or bronchitis-like illness. RSV outbreaks usually occur between October and May, with a peak in January and February. The most severe RSV infections occur in young infants, especially premature infants with underlying lung problems. RSV is a highly contagious disease, as nearly every child experiences at least one RSV infection by two years of age. Half of all children infected during their first year of life will be re-infected with RSV in their second year of life. The RSV re-infection rate is even higher in infants attending day-care centers. The most common symptoms of an RSV infection are fever, wheezing, coughing, and chest congestion.

What is the link between RSV and asthma? Several decades ago, researchers found that more than 50 percent of children with RSV-bronchiolitis had further episodes of wheezing, and were twice as likely to develop asthma later on in childhood. RSV was believed to trigger several years or even a lifetime of asthma. Now it appears that the RSV virus itself does not trigger asthma unless it attacks infants or young children with other asthma risk factors, such as a high IgE level, eczema or food allergies, a family history of allergy or asthma, or exposure to tobacco smoke.

Viral Infections in Adults

Under certain circumstances, adult viral infections favor the development of asthma. Adult hospital admission rates for asthma are highest when children return to school, mirroring the trends seen in childhood asthma. This explains why many adults develop asthma for the first time in their lives after a simple viral respiratory infection. Such respiratory infections may also reactivate latent asthma that had been present in childhood. Taken together, these observations strongly support the concept that the airway response to viral infections and allergens may share common pathways.

The clinical manifestations of the upper and lower airway response to viral and bacterial infections are dependent on multiple factors including age, sex, family history, and allergen and passive smoke exposure. The interrelationship between viral infections, allergic disease, sinus infections, and asthma is especially intriguing. The anecdotal evidence supporting the link between respiratory viral infections and episodes of asthma in adults is less well established. Few studies have tested the concept that viral infections trigger acute asthma in adults.

Mycoplasma and Chlamydia Infection

Interesting research by Dr. Richard Martin from National Jewish Hospital in Denver, Colorado, discovered that nearly 60 percent of the asthma patients he studied harbored mycoplasma bacteria in their lungs. Martin initiated this study after he found this mycoplasma bacteria in the lungs of a twenty-four-year-old woman with severe lifelong asthma who dramatically improved after she was placed on the antibiotic clarithromycin. Over the next five years she took this antibiotic on a daily basis and was able to stop oral prednisone and resume normal day-to-day activities. Dr. Martin then postulated that people with persistent asthma might be chronically infected with mycoplasma bacteria.

This story is not unlike the discovery by two Australian physicians, who found that their patients with chronic peptic ulcer disease were infected with a bacteria called heliobacter pylori. Dr. Martin is now conducting a five-year study to determine if chronic mycoplasma infection causes asthma. This theory brings up an intriguing question. Another type of infectious agent, chlamydia pneumonaie, may play a role in asthma. Chlamydia pneumonaie, an unusual human pathogen discovered in 1986, is a unique organism that strikes both birds and humans and causes a variety of infections, including bronchitis and pneumonia. One form of the bird-borne chlamydia disease causes a severe form of pneumonia in humans called psittacosis. Chlamydia also causes blindness (trachoma), infertility, and chronic urinary tract infections. Most human chlamydia infections are low-grade infections that can go undetected for months or years.

Some researchers believe that chronic infection with chlamydia may be linked to asthma and COPD. Doctors can test for chlamydia and, when indicated, administer appropriate antibiotics. These findings need additional research before asthma specialists recommend widespread use of antibiotics in all people with chronic asthma. However, I believe that a six- to eight-week trial of an appropriate antibiotic is indicated in people with severe persistent asthma, as it may be years before we have a valid answer to the question of whether or not chronic bacterial infections, such as mycoplasma or chlamydia, cause asthma.

New Theories

The hygiene hypothesis proposes that exposure to naturally acquired infections or even parasites in infancy and early childhood may protect against asthma. For the past thirty years, I have been telling my patients that the existence of allergies predisposes them to the common cold.

The evidence to support this statement is weak at best. Nevertheless, there is agreement among asthma specialists that pre-existing inflammation in the lung accentuates the effects of viral infections.

University of California investigators inoculated allergic subjects with a nasal allergen before deliberately infecting them with a common cold virus. They expected to prove that a pre-existing allergy would worsen the effects of the common cold. Much to their surprise they found just the opposite. Pre-exposure to an offending allergen delayed the onset of cold symptoms and reduced the duration of the cold. Thus, pre-existing allergy may in some way protect against or reduce the symptoms of the common cold. At the present time, there is no final answer as to the protective or harmful role played by viral, bacterial, or parasitic infections in asthma. It is probably a two-way street. In other words, certain viral infections like the common cold and RSV may lead to asthma, whereas other naturally acquired infections may prevent allergy and asthma.

CHAPTER NINE

Drug Therapy and Asthma

The drugs used to treat asthma have different effects. Bronchodilating or relieving drugs, like the beta-agonists and theophylline, open up or dilate the bronchial tubes. While these drugs prevent or relieve the symptoms of the early phase of asthma, they have little or no effect on the late phase or inflammatory response. The controlling or anti-inflammatory drugs like cromolyn, cortisone, and the new leukotriene inhibitors do not relieve acute asthma symptoms. They prevent or control the late-phase inflammatory response.

The Relieving or Bronchodilating Drugs

Beta-agonist drugs stimulate a part of our nervous system called the sympathetic nervous system. Drugs that act directly on a receptor in the nervous system called the beta receptor are called beta-agonist drugs. The sympathetic system controls the tone of the bronchial tubes by counteracting the constricting impulses of the opposing cholinergic or bronchoconstricting system. The sympathetic system has three types of receptors, or signal boxes, that regulate heart rate, blood pressure, and bronchial tone. The alpha receptor tightens muscles and increases the production of mucus. The beta-1 receptor increases heart rate and blood pressure. The beta-2 receptor is the bronchodilator receptor that relaxes smooth muscle and decreases mucus production. Older asthma drugs, like adrenaline and ephedrine, acted on all three receptors. When you got a shot of adrenaline or took ephedrine, you stopped wheezing because of the drug's effect on the beta-2 receptor. However, stimulation of the alpha and beta-1 receptors often caused tremors and an increase in pulse rate or blood pressure.

Asthma Aerosols

These shortcomings led to the search for an ideal asthma drug, one that would selectively stimulate the all-important beta-2 receptor. Aerosol or inhaled drugs are preferred over oral preparations for several reasons. After a drug is swallowed, it is absorbed into the blood stream and circulates to all organs in the body. One must take a relatively large amount of drug to deliver a small dose to a selected target organ like the lung. The drug is also transported to other organs and causes unwanted side effects. The shortcomings of oral drugs prompted researchers to look for drugs that could be delivered directly to the lung.

The first drug to be successfully used as an asthma aerosol was adrenaline, a relatively weak bronchodilator with a brief duration of action. Adrenaline also caused an increase in blood pressure and heart rate, as it stimulated both the alpha and beta-1 receptor. This primitive asthma aerosol is still available in a popular over-the-counter (OTC) drug called Primatene Mist. The next aerosol to be developed was isoproterenol, a more powerful drug than adrenaline. This drug, sold under the brand names of Medihaler-Iso and Isuprel Mistometer, was the most widely used asthma aerosol from 1950 to 1970. Like adrenaline, it had a short duration of action and a tendency to increase heart rate and blood pressure. In 1961, English investigators announced the discovery of a new beta-agonist drug, called metaproterenol or Alupent. This new product was a more selective beta-2 agonist that lasted longer and was less likely to increase blood pressure or heart rate. Over the next twenty years, many other effective beta-2 agonist drugs would be developed, including terbutaline (Brethine), bitolterol (Tornalate), pirbuterol (Maxair), and albuterol (Proventil or Ventolin). Albuterol is now the most effective and widely used short-acting bronchodilator. In addition to reversing acute asthma, albuterol can prevent and relieve exercise-induced asthma. In 1992, salmeterol (Serevent), a longer-acting beta-agonist drug with a twelve-hour duration of action, became available. The newest long-acting beta-agonist, formoterol (Foradil), became available in 2001.

Beta-agonist drugs are administered by mouth, by injection, intravenously, or by inhalation. The preferred route of administration is by inhalation or aerosol due to a rapid onset of action and less risk of side effects. Short-acting beta-agonists are front-line drugs for relieving acute asthma and preventing exercise-induced asthma. Due to their limited duration of action, they are not well suited for maintenance bronchodilator therapy. In most instances, beta-agonists are administered via a metered dose inhaler or MDI or dry powdered inhalers or DPIs. If you experience difficulty using an inhaler, you might benefit from using spacers or holding chambers. Sometimes young children and older adults will require a nebulizer to administer their beta-agonist drug.

Side Effects of the Beta-Agonists

Potential side effects of the beta-agonists include an increase in heart rate and blood pressure and a transient fall in blood oxygen levels in people with acute asthma. This fall in oxygen level is not considered to be an important problem, but oxygen levels should be monitored when treating acute asthma. Other common side effects of beta-agonist therapy are jitteriness or tremors—the result of stimulation of the skeletal muscle beta-1 receptor. The two most commonly used over-the-counter inhalers that contain epinephrine, Primatene and Bronkaid

Mist, continue to sell millions of canisters per year. Both these drugs increase pulse rate, raise blood pressure, and cause tremors. They also have a very short duration of action—about twenty minutes. The biggest risk of these inhalers is that they lull asthmatics into a false sense of security that prevents them from seeking the proper medical care as doctors have no way to monitor refills or detect excess use of the OTC products.

Long-Acting Beta-Agonists

Over the past ten years, selective beta-agonists with a longer duration of action have come into play. Currently, there are two long-acting compounds available, formoterol (Foradil Aerolixer) and salmeterol (Serevent). These drugs are administered via a metered-dose or dry powder inhaler. Formoterol and salmeterol have a bronchodilating effect of over twelve hours, and are more potent than albuterol. Dr. Ann Woolcock studied poorly controlled asthmatics taking inhaled cortisone drugs and found that adding salmeterol (Serevent), while not increasing the daily dose of the inhaled cortisone drug, had better results—less nighttime wheezing, improved pulmonary function tests, less need for rescue medication—than doubling the daily dose of their inhaled cortisone.

There is no doubt that the introduction of long-acting beta-2 agonists represents a significant milestone in asthma therapy. It is now generally agreed these drugs are indicated in people who fail to respond to inhaled cortisone drugs alone. However, some studies have shown that daily use of a long-acting beta-agonist may mask inflammation and delay one's awareness of worsening asthma.

In January 2003, GlaxoSmithKline (GSK) notified the FDA that it was stopping a large study on its long-acting bronchodilator, Serevent. After enrolling 26,000 asthmatics in this study, GSK found a small increase in the number of near-fatal and fatal asthma attacks in people on salmeterol, especially in African-Americans who were using this drug alone to control their asthma. GSK subsequently put a "black box" warning on this drug that advises people not to use this drug as a single entity. Thus, anyone using a long-acting beta-agonist must also take an inhaled cortisone drug on a regular basis. GlaxoSmithKline's drug, Advair, a combination of an inhaled cortisone (Flovent) and a long-acting beta-agonist (Serevent), has been a beneficial product for people who require both of these asthma drugs.

Third-Generation Beta-Agonists

Through clever pharmacology, research chemists have been able to alter the basic structure of the older beta-agonist drug albuterol. One compound, levalbuterol (Xopenex), possesses desirable bronchodilating characteristics, yet does not cause undesirable side effects like tremors and increased heart rate. Xopenex has been shown to have an excellent safety record and duration of action of up to eight hours. Now available only as an aerosol for nebulizers, Xopenex manufacturers are developing a hand-held inhaler which should be available in the near future.

The Beta-Agonist Debate

The debate over the role of the inhaled beta-agonist drugs in asthma is a long and controversial one, dating back to the late 1960s when asthma mortality increased in England and Wales. British investigators found that the increase in asthma deaths in England followed the introduction of a potent beta-agonist drug, called Isoproterenol Forte. In 1967, the United Kingdom issued a warning on this product. Sudden and unexplained asthma deaths in young people were tied to excess use of this beta-agonist aerosol. After Isoproterenol Forte was removed from OTC sales, asthma mortality rates significantly declined.

In the early 1980s, another asthma mortality epidemic in young asthmatics was reported in New Zealand. These reports implied that overuse of the beta-agonist drugs played a role in asthma deaths. A

New Zealand Asthma Mortality Study Group thoroughly reviewed 271 asthma deaths and could only identify nine cases where excess use of beta-agonists triggered an asthma death. This report emphasized the risks of under-utilization of treatment and a delay in seeking appropriate treatment during relapsing asthma.

However, many asthma specialists disagreed with these conclusions. Dr. Neil Pearce from Wellington, New Zealand, proposed that that introduction of a long-acting and more potent beta-agonist, fenoterol, was the cause of the New Zealand asthma death epidemic, as the increase in asthma deaths coincided with the introduction of fenoterol to New Zealand. Dr. Malcolm Sears added additional fuel to this fire in December 1990. Sears's well-designed, placebo-controlled study evaluated sixty-four asthmatics for six months. One group took their inhaled beta-agonist (fenoterol) on a regular basis; the other group used it strictly on an as-needed or on-demand basis. The as-needed or on-demand group had fewer bouts of nighttime asthma, less need for prednisone, lower bronchial reactivity, and better peak flow rates than people who used their beta-agonist on a regular basis. Dr. Sears concluded that round-the-clock inhalation of a beta-agonist drug was associated with poorer control of asthma compared with people who only used their inhaler on demand or only as needed. One attractive explanation for the poor asthma control in the round-the-clock users was that people using beta-agonists regularly experience higher exposures to allergens and asthma triggers. Sears strongly recommended that inhaled beta-agonist drugs should be used only on demand to relieve acute asthma and that the practice of regular round-the-clock inhalations of beta-agonists should be discarded.

Sears's paper generated heated discussions within the medical profession. Experts pointed out that the findings of this study should not be applied to all beta-agonists, as fenoterol was a much more potent beta-agonist than the shorter-acting beta-agonists like albuterol. A Canadian survey by Dr. Walter Spitzer of McGill University in 1992 examined the medical records of 12,031 asthmatics who took asthma drugs between 1978 and 1987. Spitzer found that the forty-four people who died from asthma used twice as many inhalers as those who did not die from asthma. People using two inhaler canisters per month were more than twice as likely to die from asthma.

There were several possible explanations for the association between beta-agonist use and asthma deaths. People with severe asthma are more likely to use more asthma inhalers, beta-agonists have an adverse effect on the cardiovascular system, or beta-agonists may open up the airways too much and increase bronchial hyperreactivity. Lastly, over-reliance on beta-agonists misled people into thinking their asthma was under control, which caused them to delay seeking proper asthma care.

Critics of this report pointed out that many Canadians were using fenoterol (Berotec), a drug not available in the United States. This is the same drug that alarmed investigators in New Zealand in the 1980s. Concerns generated by this report created justifiable anxiety among asthmatic people and their families. The two major allergy organizations in the United States, the American College of Allergy, Asthma and Immunology and the American Academy of Allergy, Asthma and Immunology, issued press releases stating that there was not enough data to justify sweeping changes in the use of beta-agonist drugs.

The beta-agonist debate raises one important question. Should asthmatics take beta-agonist drugs on a round-the-clock or only on an as-needed basis? I believe the answer to this question falls into a gray zone. Inhaled beta-agonist drugs are still the most effective drugs for relieving acute asthma attack and preventing exercise-induced asthma. Many asthma care providers, including myself, now recommend using inhaled beta-agonists only on an as-needed basis in stable patients with normal peak flow rates. People with unstable asthma and wide fluctuations in peak flow rates may require regular use of long-acting bronchodilators, particularly in the morning or at bedtime.

The Theophylline Drugs

In 1859, an article in Scotland's *Edinburgh Medical Journal* stated, "One of the commonest and best reputed remedies of asthma, and one that in many cases is more effective than others, is strong tea or coffee." Unfortunately, this sage advice was ignored for more than fifty years, until German and American research teams set out to determine why asthmatics stopped wheezing when they drank strong tea or coffee. In 1888, the disclosure that caffeine was a mild bronchodilator led to the discovery of the caffeine-like drug called theophylline. Boehringer and Sons began industrial production of theophylline in Germany at the turn of the century. Initially, American doctors were slow to accept theophylline, until a 1938 report in the *Journal of the American Medical Association* noted that people with asthma experienced marked relief after receiving an intravenous injection of a form of theophylline, called aminophylline. Oral forms of theophylline were then developed. However, theophylline had many drawbacks, including a bitter taste and a tendency to cause nausea and vomiting. This problem was partially solved when chemists added other drugs to the theophylline drugs to improve its taste and reduce side effects.

The Three-In-One Drugs

In 1940, a *New England Journal of Medicine* report by Dr. Ethan Allen Brown cited Dr. Brown's success in clinical trials with a new oral medication called Tedral, a combination of three drugs in one tablet—theophylline, ephedrine, and phenobarbital. This combination drug and others like it became the backbone of outpatient asthma therapy for the next thirty years. These drugs had several disadvantages. Doses of each individual drug could not be increased separately. For example, people requiring a higher dose of theophylline also had to take more oral ephedrine, a potent stimulant that caused insomnia, tremors, and heart palpitations.

Today, these outdated fixed-combination drugs would not receive approval from the FDA. The glaring deficiencies of the combination drugs were ignored until 1972, when Dr. Elliot Ellis from National Jewish Hospital in Denver urged doctors to use theophylline as a single drug that allowed each patient's dose to be individualized. These efforts sparked another revolution in asthma therapy, leading to the development of pure, more effective theophylline compounds. The first single theophylline preparations were short-acting drugs that only lasted a few hours. Innovative alterations in theophylline tablet and capsule design produced longer-acting drugs that allowed once- or twice-a-day dosing. Children metabolize, or use up, theophylline much more rapidly than adults. A fifty-pound child may require more theophylline on the basis of body weight than a two-hundred-pound adult. Smokers need more theophylline than non-smokers, and elderly asthmatics often require less theophylline. After researchers developed a simple blood test, called a theophylline blood level, to determine if people were taking too little or too much theophylline, doses could be precisely tailored to individual needs for the first time in asthma therapy.

Theophylline Interactions and Side Effects

Different drugs prescribed for different medical conditions may interact when they combine in the body. For example, when an asthmatic on oral theophylline develops an infection and requires the antibiotic erythromycin, the combination of both theophylline and erythromycin may cause significant problems. When these drugs are taken at the same time, erythromycin slows down the rate at which theophylline is metabolized, which in effect doubles the amount of theophylline in the body. Thus, a normal dose of theophylline acts like a double dose when taken along with erythromycin. This drug interaction causes a theophylline overdose. Many other drugs interact with theophylline, including the ulcer drug cimetadine (Tagamet) and blood pressure-migraine medicine propranolol (Inderal). Some viral infections also double the effect of theophylline.

Long-term use of theophylline is usually no more hazardous than the daily consumption of tea or coffee. About one in every ten people may develop nausea, loss of appetite, or vomiting. Some children become hyperactive or develop learning problems, as theophylline has been found to decrease attention span and concentration in some people. Additional theophylline side effects include headache, insomnia, and jitteriness. Most of these side effects are due to the caffeine-like properties of theophylline. People who cannot tolerate coffee or tea cannot usually take theophylline. As one of my theophylline-intolerant patients aptly stated, "When I take theophylline, I feel like I've overdosed on coffee." The minor theophylline side effects that occur soon after starting treatment often subside after a few days of therapy, or are eliminated by taking the drug with food or after meals. Sometimes, a dose reduction is necessary, and occasionally theophylline must be discontinued altogether. Fortunately, the major toxic reactions caused by high blood theophylline levels—vomiting of blood, mental confusion, and seizures—are rare.

Theophylline therapy continues to have its ups and downs. Once the first-line drug or mainstay of asthma therapy in both the doctor's office and the emergency room, theophylline has been relegated to the fourth line of asthma defense. The reasons for this demotion are twofold. Theophylline has many side effects and a narrow dosing range between effectiveness and toxicity. Secondly, the availability of safer and more effective asthma medications like inhaled cortisone, long-acting beta-agonists, and the new leukotriene modifiers have pushed theophylline to the back of the bus. Should theophylline be kicked off the bus altogether? My answer to this question is no. Theophylline is an effective drug for people with stubborn nocturnal asthma. Once-a-day theophylline drugs may be quite helpful in elderly people with mild asthma. Theophylline may also turn the tide in severe asthma that is unresponsive to inhaled cortisone drugs, long-acting beta-agonists, and the leukotriene modifiers.

I would not be surprised if newer and safer theophylline-like drugs actually make a comeback in the next few years. Recent studies have shown that low-dose theophylline has anti-inflammatory activity. One asthma guru, Dr. Peter Barnes from London, has stated that theophylline drugs are more effective in severe asthma than the new leukotriene modifiers. To minimize side effects, theophylline treatment should be initiated with low doses, and the final dose should be carefully adjusted. People on maintenance theophylline therapy should have their blood level monitored once or twice a year. I usually maintain a theophylline blood level between five and ten. Such a level minimizes the chances for a drug interaction due to viral illness or the presence of another drug that may produce a theophylline level over thirty, the level at which most major toxic reactions occur.

The Anticholinergic Drugs

Bronchial tube smooth-muscle tone is kept in balance by the opposing actions of the sympathetic and parasympathetic nervous system. The bronchodilating drugs act on the sympathetic side of the system. What about drugs that block the opposing or cholinergic system? This system is the excitatory part of the nervous system, and any drug that acts here would have to inhibit or block this side of the nervous system. In fact, these so-called anticholinergic drugs have been used for centuries to treat asthma.

Derivatives of belladonna and stramonium were first used as burning powders and asthma cigarettes and cigars. R.R. Schiffman recognized the potential of atropine-like drugs seventy years ago, when he advocated smoking Schiffman's Asthma Cigarettes for the treatment of asthma. These cigarettes were derived from the leaves of the thorne apple tree that contained stramonium, an atropine-like drug. Naturally the risks of inhaling stramonium leaves far outweighed any potential benefit of these asthma-inhibiting cigars or cigarettes.

Atropine, the first cholinergic drug to be synthesized, is routinely given to people prior to surgery to dry up mucus secretions during anesthesia and surgery. A renewed interest in the potential benefit of anticholinergic drugs in respiratory diseases led to the development of an inhaled cholinergic drug, called ipratropium bromide (Atrovent). Inhaled ipratropium bromide owes its safety to the fact that it is poorly absorbed. While it is not as potent a bronchodilator as the beta-agonist drugs, it may be helpful in asthmatics who produce a lot of mucus or have chronic bronchitis from cigarette smoking. It can also be used to treat acute asthma along with a short-acting beta-agonist to help get asthma under control more quickly. One product that combines both ipratropium and albuterol (Combivent) is very helpful in asthmatics with chronic bronchitis and excess mucus production. The newest anticholinergic drug, Spiriva (topraproprium), appears promising as it can be given just once a day by a clearly designed HandiHaler device. While it is mainly indicated for COPD patients, some asthmatics who produce a lot of sputum may benefit from it. Spiriva's most common side effect is a dry mouth that often resolves over time.

CHAPTER TEN

The Controlling Drugs

The last chapter reviewed the role of the reliever drugs or bronchodilators in asthma; now we discuss the asthma-controller drugs.

Cromolyn Sodium

Cromolyn sodium or Intal was the first controller drug to be developed. Dr. Roger Altounyan discovered this unique preparation. Dr. Altounyan, a brilliant English scientist and lifelong asthma sufferer, became interested in a derivative of an Egyptian herbal plant called khellin. Altounyan suspected that khellin might have an anti-asthmatic effect, as it was a muscle relaxant used in ancient times to relieve intestinal colic. While studying khellin, Altounyan volunteered to be a human guinea pig. He deliberately inhaled derivatives of khellin to determine if they could block his asthma attacks.

Several years and approximately two thousand asthma attacks later, Altounyan isolated a safe and effective asthma-preventing compound called cromolyn sodium or Intal. Since cromolyn was poorly absorbed by the intestinal tract, Altounyan figured out a way to get the cromolyn powder into the lung. Drawing on his World War II RAF flying experience,

Altounyan developed an ingenious propeller-driven device called the Spinhaler to deliver Intal powder into the lung. This unique device was the forerunner of today's dry powder inhalers.

A Closer Look at Cromolyn

In some way that is not fully understood, cromolyn inhibits the release of mediators from the mast cell. Cromolyn is the only asthma drug capable of blocking both the early and late phases of the asthmatic response. Cromolyn was subjected to more than a thousand clinical trials throughout the world. The largest American study reviewed its effects on 252 people. Seventy percent of these study patients improved. More importantly, 50 percent who needed oral cortisone to control their asthma were able to taper or discontinue their oral cortisone drug.

Initial fears that this relatively unknown powder could harm the lung were unfounded, as were the theoretical concerns that cromolyn, being an anti-allergy drug, could injure the immune system. I have never seen a skin rash or any significant side effect from cromolyn, which I have used for nearly twenty years in hundreds of patients. In my experience cromolyn side effects are very rare. It could be the safest drug in all of medicine.

Who Benefits from Cromolyn?

Cromolyn works best in children and some adults with mild, persistent allergic asthma. It prevents asthma triggered by an animal exposure or exercise. Sometimes cromolyn will relieve a stubborn case of hidden or cough-variant asthma that does not respond to other asthma medicines. Cromolyn should not be used to treat acute asthma. Because cromolyn does not work as well in more severe or non-allergic asthma, pulmonary specialists are less enthusiastic about this drug.

Cromolyn is a valuable drug in treating mild, persistent asthma, especially in young children. The fact that the cromolyn capsule and Intal Spinhaler was too complicated a delivery method for many infants and young children led to the development of an Intal solution that could be administered by a nebulizer. In that era the Intal solution represented a major advance in asthma therapy for infants and young children. The developers of cromolyn went one step further when they released an Intal metered-dose inhaler. Cromolyn is not just an asthma drug. It is also an effective drug for allergic rhinitis (Nasalcrom) and eye allergy (Opticrom). The major disadvantage of cromolyn is that it must be given three to four times a day on a regular basis. I now use cromolyn to prevent exercise-induced asthma or when there is a problem with the inhaled cortisone drugs.

The Cortisone Drugs

Before discussing the role of cortisone drugs in asthma, we must review the basic function of our adrenal gland. The adrenal gland, a small gland located behind the kidneys, produces three types of cortisone hormones. The first group, the mineralocorticoid hormones, regulates the body's salt balance. The second group, the anabolic steroids, controls growth, muscle mass, and sexual features. The third group, the glucocorticoids, regulates levels of sugar, fat, and protein in the body, and fights inflammation. This anti-inflammatory effect is what makes the inhaled cortisone drugs the most effective of all asthma medications.

Even though all three cortisone compounds are made in the adrenal gland, the corticosteroids used in the treatment of asthma have no anabolic effects (they do not increase hair growth or muscle mass), and they have little effect on the body's salt balance. Corticosteroids act on virtually every cell and gland involved in asthma, including the mucus glands, macrophages, smooth muscle cells, mast cells, T-cells or lymphocytes, and the eosinophils.

After cortisone was chemically isolated from human adrenal glands in 1948, the results of early clinical trials in asthma were spectacular. The sickest of asthmatics stopped wheezing for the first time in years. Doctors thought that the cure for asthma and a host of other diseases, like arthritis, had finally arrived. Initial enthusiasm for cortisone waned when it became apparent that taking oral cortisone over a long period had devastating side effects, including adrenal gland suppression, slow wound healing, excess weight gain, easy bruising, brittle bones (osteoporosis), eye cataracts, and growth retardation in children. When it was discovered that many unacceptable side effects of daily oral cortisone could be avoided by taking cortisone every other day, "alternate-day therapy" became a well-accepted method for treating asthma that did not respond to the conventional asthma drugs. Alternate-day therapy allowed many severe asthmatics to stay out of the hospital and lead relatively normal lives. Prednisone and prednisolone (Medrol) became the drugs of choice in alternate-day therapy, as they have a very short half-life. Even so, alternate-day therapy was not totally risk-free, as many patients still developed serious side effects with long-term cortisone alternate-day therapy.

Cortisone Inhalers to the Rescue

The dangers posed by daily or alternate-day therapy prompted a search for safer cortisone drugs. People needed drugs that could be delivered in relatively low doses with a metered dose inhaler. In 1951, inhaled cortisone was suspended in saline. This was followed in 1960 by release of the Decadron Respihaler, a potent adrenal-suppressive drug with severe cortisone side effects. Asthma specialists can thank their dermatology colleagues for the development of the first safe and effective inhaled cortisone drugs. Beclomethasone was developed from a topical spray used on the skin in eczema sufferers.

In the late 1970s two inhaled beclomethasone cortisone drugs, Vanceril and Beclovent, were introduced for asthma. In my opinion the development of this class of asthma drugs was and still remains the most important advance in asthma therapy in my career. Clinical experience with inhaled cortisone drugs over the past two decades has demonstrated their superiority in controlling chronic asthma in all ages.

The five inhaled cortisone drugs currently available in the United States are beclomethasone (Q-Var), flunisolide (AeroBid), triamcinolone (Azmacort), fluticasone (Flovent), and budesonide (Pulmicort). Flunisolide and triamcinolone were approved for use in 1984, and the two more potent cortisone inhalers, fluticasone and budesonide, became available in the 1990s. Another inhaled cortisone preparation, mometasone (Asmanex), should become available sometime in the near future. The lack of a nebulized cortisone drug for infants and young children was solved after budesonide (Pulmicort) became available in a nebulized solution called Pulmicort Respules.

A new and novel combination drug was approved by the FDA in 2000. This drug, called Advair Diskus, which is delivered by a breath-actuated powder device, combines a long-acting beta-agonist, salmeterol (Serevent), and the inhaled cortisone drug fluticasone (Flovent). This combination drug can be given as one puff once or twice a day to children and adults who need both a relieving and a controlling asthma drug on a daily basis. The convenience of having two medications in one and needing only two puffs per day has dramatically improved compliance.

The favorable results gained by more than twenty-five years of experience with these drugs imply that their risk-benefit ratio favors the use of these most potent asthma-controlling drugs. Before these drugs became available in the 1970s, I had at least two dozen patients in my practice with severe asthma who could only be controlled with alternate-day prednisone. Thanks to the availability of the inhaled cortisone drugs, very few of my patients need long-term daily or alternate-day prednisone therapy.

Choosing an Inhaled Cortisone Drug

Choosing one inhaled cortisone formulation over another is difficult. Health-care providers have a wide choice of several preparations with varying strengths and dosing schedules. The best way to compare different inhaled corticosteroids is to look at their therapeutic index, which is the ratio between desired and undesired clinical effects. The higher the therapeutic index, the better the risk-benefit ratio. Undesired effects are related to the amount of inhaled drug that is absorbed into the circulation and delivered to other body organs.

Older inhaled cortisone drugs are more readily absorbed once the particles are swallowed, whereas the absorption from the newer inhaled cortisone drugs like fluticasone (Flovent) and budesonide (Pulmicort) comes from the inhaled fraction that enters the lung. Studies have concluded that all the inhaled cortisone drugs have side effects when given in high enough doses. No data exists to allow one to determine the superiority of one drug over another. Sometimes it is necessary to take the questions of cost, convenience, patient preference, or HMO and insurance coverage into consideration.

In summary, the inhaled cortisone drugs are the most effective long-term control medications for asthma. They carry less risk than other drugs such as oral prednisone, theophylline, or the long-acting beta-agonist drugs. When the inhaled corticosteroids are compared head to head to all other asthma drugs, such as cromolyn, long-acting beta-agonists, theophylline, and the newer leukotriene modifiers, the inhaled cortisone drugs always come out on top.

While serious side effects are uncommon, parents of asthmatic children and adults with asthma should be informed that these drugs are not completely risk-free, especially when used in higher doses. For those people who require higher doses to control asthma, the potential for systemic effects are still less when compared to the complications in untreated asthma and the need for frequent bursts of prednisone. One must carefully weigh the risk-benefit ratio of the inhaled cortisone drugs and constantly try to "step-down" doses to achieve the lowest possible dose that maintains normal or near-normal lung function and quality of life. The 1997 NHLBI Guidelines identify inhaled cortisone drugs as the preferred treatment of asthma. To date, no other asthma medication has been shown to be as effective as these inhaled cortisone drugs.

In December 2003, the American College of Chest Physicians, the American Academy of Allergy, Asthma and Immunology and the American College of Allergy, Asthma and Immunology issued a consensus statement in the journal *Chest* that stated, "inhaled cortisone or ICS therapy has been the gold standard for asthma therapy for the past twenty years. However, since the inception of such therapy, physicians have been concerned about side effects, particularly in children, women and the elderly." An expert panel from these three organizations reviewed 108 studies of adult and pediatric asthma that looked at the side effects of ICS therapy. The panel concluded that evidence supports the conclusion that the clinical effectiveness of ICS therapy decidedly outweighs the proven risks. One additional and unexpected benefit of these drugs is found in a recent Canadian study that found that adults taking an inhaled cortisone drug had a decreased risk of heart attacks.

I agree with this consensus statement that inhaled cortisone drugs are the "gold standard" or cornerstone of asthma therapy. Over the past few years, doctors have noticed a trend: Adults and children are more likely to use cortisone drugs early on, even in cases of mild, persistent asthma. The pros and cons of this "treat early and often" approach will be discussed in chapter twenty-two, when I review the NHLBI treatment guidelines for asthma.

The Prednisone Pulse

Most savvy health-care consumers are aware of the inherent dangers posed by the long-term use of daily or alternate-day oral cortisone or prednisone. However, many are not aware that the cortisone drugs used in asthma are vastly different from the anabolic steroids that athletes use to build up their muscle mass. Such anabolic steroids are synthetic sex hormones that cause growth retardation, severe liver damage, psychological problems, and other serious harm. Unfortunately, many people (and some doctors) have "steroid phobia," which means that they are unduly apprehensive about using prednisone for short periods of time in unstable asthma.

Physicians like myself who completed medical training in the 1970s were taught that oral prednisone took a long time to exert its effect, and it should only be used in very severe or life-threatening asthma attacks. Fortunately, such erroneous concepts have been recognized, and the pendulum has actually swung to the other extreme. Asthma specialists now mandate the administration of a short burst of cortisone or prednisone to any patient with moderate or severe asthma who is experiencing an acute asthma relapse.

The oral cortisone drug of choice in acute asthma is prednisone or prednisolone (Prelone or Orapred) in children. These drugs have a shorter half-life or length of duration of action than other oral cortisone preparations. Studies have shown the short-term use of oral prednisone is both safe and effective. A beneficial effect can sometimes be seen as early as three to four hours after the initial dose of oral prednisone. The prompt use of a well-timed pulse of prednisone reduces the need for acute emergency visits and hospitalization in both children and adults. In my opinion, it is the only drug that may prevent a near-fatal or fatal asthma attack. Emergency room studies have shown that prompt use of the prednisone pulse lowers the likelihood of an asthma relapse.

People who receive a prednisone pulse are more likely to have normal lung functions a week or two after taking prednisone. In my experience, many people remain stable for weeks or months after just one short burst of prednisone. The prednisone doses used in acute asthma are strictly empirical, as there is little dose-response data dealing with cortisone and asthma. Since toxicity is directly related to duration of treatment, not dosage, most asthma specialists choose a high enough dose to be at or near the top of the dose-response curve. Most children and young adults respond to an initial dose of 30 to 60 milligrams of prednisone a day, followed by a seven- to fourteen-day tapering dose. While some asthma specialists prefer to give full doses for four to five days and then abruptly stop prednisone, recent studies favor a gradual tapering of the drug.

People with severe asthma may need two to three weeks of prednisone. Short-term prednisone therapy is a very safe and effective way to stabilize asthma that is out of control and not responding to the other asthma drugs. Studies in children have demonstrated that the prednisone pulse can be safely administered up to four to five times a year.

I will prescribe a prednisone pulse to the following groups of relapsing asthmatics:

- Acutely ill people with previous hospitalizations or a history of life-threatening asthma
- Relapsing patients who are overusing their cortisone aerosols or pocket inhalers
- Unstable asthmatics with poor lung function tests
- Unstable asthmatics who may be traveling or vacationing in remote areas where good medical care is unavailable

Risks of the Prednisone Pulse

Potential side effects from the prednisone pulse include slight weight gain, increased appetite, menstrual irregularities, acne flare-ups, mood changes, muscle cramps, and heartburn or indigestion. To prevent muscle cramps, drink orange juice or eat bananas, which restore potassium. To prevent heartburn, take antacids, anti-ulcer drugs, or prednisone after meals. People with tuberculosis, diabetes, high blood pressure, glaucoma, esophageal reflux, ulcers, or psychosis require closer observation when they take prednisone.

The long-term use of oral steroids has devastating side effects. Some of the more serious complications that will be discussed in the next chapter include adrenal gland failure, cataracts, decreased bone mass (osteoporosis), decreased growth rate in children, high blood pressure, elevated blood sugar, and easy bruising. These more serious side effects are seen in those people who take higher-than-normal alternate-day prednisone doses, usually over 30 milligrams every other day. Such side effects do not usually occur with the short-term use of prednisone or with conventional doses of the cortisone inhalers.

People who do require alternate-day steroids should take their dose in the morning every other day. This allows the adrenal gland time to work on its own on the off day. Prednisone is the least expensive of all asthma drugs, and comes in liquid and tablet forms in various dosing strengths. Two liquid preparations, Prelone and Orapred, are very helpful for children and adults who cannot swallow tablets.

Keeping Time with the Circadian Rhythm

Many of our bodily functions like blood pressure, temperature, lung function, and hormone output cycle through predictable patterns every twenty-four hours. This is called circadian rhythm. Two important hormones, epinephrine and cortisone, peak at 9 a.m., decrease slightly in the daytime, and fall to their lowest levels in the middle of the night. Some of the chemicals that trigger asthma peak in the middle of the night. This explains why many asthmatics are prone to nocturnal wheezing. Thus, in some people the timing of drug dosing becomes all-important. For example, taking a medicine at bedtime may reduce morning symptoms. Using your inhaled cortisone medication may prevent nighttime asthma if taken between 3 and 5 p.m.

Steroid-Resistant Asthma

A small group of people with severe, persistent asthma will not respond to high doses of inhaled or oral cortisone drugs. The term doctors apply to this group of people is steroid-resistant asthma. Several factors that typify people with steroid-resistant asthma include a longer duration of symptoms, low morning peak flow rates, and increased bronchial hyperresponsiveness. Steroid-resistant asthma poses a challenging problem for asthma specialists. Early identification of this form of asthma is important, not only to improve asthma control but also to avoid excessive and often debilitating cortisone side effects in people who are not benefiting from cortisone. Confounding factors such as GERD, vocal cord dysfunction, sinus disease, poor compliance or adherence with medications, and psychosocial factors should be addressed prior to categorizing a patient as a steroid-resistant asthmatic. People with true steroid-resistant asthma should be considered candidates for more sophisticated anti-inflammatory asthma drugs such as cyclosporin, methotrexate, gold, dapsone, hydroxychloroquine, intravenous gammaglobulin, or nebulized lidocaine.

CHAPTER ELEVEN

The Side Effects of the Cortisone Drugs

While the cortisone drugs are the most effective of all asthma medications, they also have the most potential for significant side effects. Adverse effects of cortisone include adrenal suppression, osteoporosis or bone loss, increased appetite with weight gain, development of a moon-shaped face, a buffalo hump or swelling in the back of the neck, wasting of the extremities, atrophy of the skin, excess hair growth, eye cataracts, growth retardation in children, and psychological disturbances.

Other less common complications include hypertension, peptic ulcer disease, and diabetes. Most of the side effects listed above are seen with prolonged use of the oral forms of cortisone.

The most common problems encountered with the inhaled cortisone drugs are oral thrush, or white spots on the mouth or tongue, and a form of hoarseness called dysphonia. The incidence and severity of thrush and hoarseness can be minimized by mouth rinsing with water and using a spacer device to reduce particle deposition in the mouth and throat. Sometimes mouth rinsing with an antifungal agent like mycostatin will be required to control oral thrush.

Adrenal Suppression

Our bodily functions are controlled by a group of glands in our body called the endocrine glands. These endocrine glands secrete hormones into the blood stream that deliver messages to various organs and tissues. The production of these hormones is regulated by the body's computer center—the brain's pituitary gland. This gland, the size of a hazelnut, is the most important of the endocrine glands because it programs sexual features, breast milk production, growth, and thyroid and adrenal gland function.

The paired adrenal glands are small organs located in our abdomen behind our kidneys. They produce several hormones including cortisone; androgens, or sex hormones; and adrenaline or epinephrine. These glands constantly exchange signals with the pituitary gland. When too much cortisone is circulating in our body, the pituitary gland sends out a signal to the adrenal glands that shuts down the production of cortisone.

Thus, when extra cortisone is introduced into our body, the adrenal glands stop cortisone production—this is called adrenal gland suppression. Any patient who takes an oral cortisone drug like prednisone on a daily basis for a long period of time will develop adrenal gland suppression. This risk is somewhat minimized by giving the drugs on an alternate-day basis, which allows the pituitary and adrenal gland to overcome the effects of extra cortisone on the off day when cortisone is not administered.

People with adrenal gland suppression can develop acute adrenal insufficiency during times of acute stress brought on by surgery, acute illness, or trauma. Acute adrenal insufficiency is a true medical emergency, and requires prompt diagnosis and treatment with extra doses of cortisone. All people on long-term oral cortisone should be considered to have adrenal suppression and wear a Medic-Alert bracelet that identifies them as being at risk for acute adrenal insufficiency. All adrenal-suppressed individuals should be given extra cortisone prior to any surgical procedure. Complete recovery from adrenal suppression may take six months to a year after cessation of long-term cortisone use.

Growth Retardation

The biggest controversy involving the side effects of inhaled cortisone drugs focuses on the potential of growth retardation in children. Before getting into this debate, let us review the pattern of normal childhood growth. Normal childhood growth occurs in three stages. First, there is the rapid growth of infancy and early childhood. After age two growth rates slow down and there is a more gradual increase in height—usually two to three inches per year. The rate of childhood growth dips to its lowest point in later childhood during the two- to three-year period preceding puberty.

The third and final stage of growth occurs in puberty. The timing of the growth spurt in puberty is variable and may start as early as ten years or as late as sixteen years of age. Some children, often referred to as "late bloomers," have a pronounced delay in growth in early puberty only to have a dramatic growth spurt later in adolescence.

How do cortisone drugs inhibit growth? Our adrenal glands make approximately 37 milligrams of cortisone each day, which is the equivalent of 7 milligrams of prednisone. Cortisone is a vital hormone that fine-tunes all of our bodily functions, including growth. Growth is controlled by growth hormone, produced in the pituitary gland. Extra cortisone suppresses all functions of this pituitary gland, including the production of growth hormone. The end result is a slowing of growth, as the large bones responsible for one's height are no longer stimulated to grow by growth hormone.

Clinical Studies on Growth

The rising incidence of asthma leading to the widespread use of inhaled cortisone drugs in children with asthma has created concerns about the possible effects of inhaled cortisone drugs on childhood growth. Preliminary, poorly controlled growth studies in children implied that inhaled cortisone could impair childhood growth. One study found a growth reduction of 1.4 to 1.5 centimeters, or one-third to one-half an inch per year. Another study found that there was no difference between final adult heights in those who took inhaled corticosteroids compared to control studies of those not using inhaled cortisone drugs. It appears that any growth rate reduction is limited to the first year of therapy. One other possibility is that adolescent growth spurt could overcome any early effect of the inhaled cortisone on growth.

The debate generated by these findings prompted the FDA to address this issue. In July 1998, the FDA recommended a labeling change for both nasal and inhaled cortisone drugs that stated that nasal and inhaled corticosteroids have been shown to cause a reduction in growth velocity when administered to children and adolescents and that the long-term effects on growth were unknown. This FDA announcement created an uproar, leading to a formal statement from the national organizations of asthma specialists. The statement pointed out that the FDA's labeling change did not imply that these products were unsafe, and warned against the abrupt termination of these asthma drugs. Undue alarm would be an inappropriate response, and asthma experts stressed that inhaled cortisone drugs were still the most effective medications available for treating the millions of people who suffer from asthma.

A Closer Look at New Studies

The CAMP or Childhood Asthma Management Program is an NIH-sponsored study that has tracked 1,041 children, five to twelve years of age, from 1991 to 2004 in eight asthma centers throughout the United States. Approximately one-third of the CAMP enrollees received the inhaled cortisone drug budesonide (Pulmicort), one-third got nedrocomil (Tilade), and another third took a placebo drug. The group treated with budesonide fared best. They had fewer asthma relapses, less need for prednisone, and fewer emergency visits or asthma hospitalizations. More importantly, no difference was noted in growth rates after one year of treatment with budesonide.

These findings support my own observation about inhaled cortisone drugs and growth. In the days before the inhaled cortisone drugs were available, I frequently had to use prednisone to control moderate to severe persistent asthma. It was well known at that time that asthma itself caused short stature and significant growth retardation. Major growth spurts were commonly observed after poorly controlled and very sick asthmatic children were placed on prednisone on an alternate-day basis.

My now 40-year-old son, who is 6 foot, 5 inches tall, has taken inhaled cortisone drugs since they first became available in the late 1970s. It is possible he may have been an inch or so taller if he had not used these inhaled cortisone drugs. But other than the fact he may have been able to grab more rebounds on the basketball court, he's living a better, healthier life because of cortisone drugs.

The Risk of Osteoporosis

Osteoporosis, the most common of all bone diseases, is estimated to affect 25 million individuals and result in 1.3 million fractures a year at a cost of $10 billion per year. The major risk factors for osteoporosis include sex (the rate is especially high in post-menopausal women) and race. Caucasians and Asians are more at risk for osteoporosis than blacks. Additional risk factors for osteoporosis include inadequate intake of calcium or vitamin D, lack of exercise, tobacco use, excess alcohol intake, and the use of cortisone medicines. In osteoporosis, the bones become too thin and fragile and are prone to fracture. The most common fracture sites are the wrist, back, hip, and leg bones. Osteoporosis can be classified as primary—age or sex related, or secondary— due to other illnesses or drugs.

The most common cause of secondary osteoporosis is the use of oral cortisone drugs. When extra amounts of cortisone are introduced into our body, there is a significant disruption in the delicate balance between the hormones that control bone formation and bone density. Exogenous or extra cortisone inhibits the production of sex hormones like testosterone and estrogen and lowers the rate of calcium absorption. The end result is bone loss or osteoporosis. Between 30 and 50 percent of people taking long-term oral corticosteroids will experience a bone fracture. Bone loss occurs rapidly (within six to twelve months) after beginning oral cortisone.

What is the risk for osteoporosis for people taking the inhaled cortisone drugs? Early studies on bone loss in people taking inhaled cortisone were poorly done and inconsistent. Some studies found that low to moderate doses of inhaled cortisone drugs have little effect on bone density. Pediatric studies have found no reduction in bone density in surveys of asthmatic children treated with low to intermediate doses of beclomethasone for several years. Remember—inhaled cortisone drugs are administered in microgram doses. A microgram is 1/1,000 of a gram. Thus, in most cases not enough drug enters the blood stream to affect bone metabolism. Some people, especially postmenopausal women, who take inhaled cortisone drugs have a long-term risk for osteoporosis.

The best way to minimize any potential bone loss in this higher-risk population is to use the lowest possible dose of inhaled cortisone drugs to control asthma and encourage weight-bearing exercises and adequate intake of calcium and vitamin D.

In summary, the current thinking indicates that the daily dose of the inhaled cortisone drug, not the duration of therapy, adversely affects bone density. Supplemental estrogen therapy may offset this bone-depleting effect in postmenopausal women. The gold standard for diagnosing bone loss or osteoporosis is a bone scan or bone densiometer study. This screening test should be done on high-risk candidates for osteoporosis.

Treatment of Osteoporosis

Once it has been determined that a patient has developed osteoporosis, early treatment is essential. Treatment programs include active exercise, especially gravity-dependent activities such as walking. Activities such as heavy lifting, high-impact aerobics, and contact sports are not recommended, as they may cause fractures of the hip, spine, or long bones. Medications include supplemental calcium and vitamin D. The NIH recommends a daily dose of 1,500 mg of calcium for women over age fifty not taking estrogen, and for all adults over age sixty-five. A daily dose of 1,000 mg of calcium is recommended for women age fifty to sixty-four who are taking estrogen, and for men age twenty-five to sixty-four. An adequate dose of vitamin D (400 to 800 units) is recommended to help the body absorb calcium. Additional medications that may be indicated include some of the newer anti-osteoporosis medications like Evista, Fosamax, and Didronel.

Glaucoma and Cataract Risks

Cortisone drugs have been linked to glaucoma and cataracts. The biggest risk for glaucoma occurs in people using oral cortisone drugs or topical cortisone eye drugs. It is believed that cortisone raises the pressure in the eye by impeding the outflow of the watery fluid in front of the eye. A study done at McGill University in Montreal, Canada, that assessed risk for increased eye pressure or glaucoma in nearly fifty thousand adults over age sixty-five who used inhaled or nasal corticosteroids found that there was no risk for people using low to medium doses of inhaled or nasal corticosteroids, but the risk for glaucoma was 44 percent higher in people taking higher doses of inhaled cortisone.

The development of eye cataracts is another potential complication of chronic cortisone use. The cataracts, while usually small, can at times impair vision and require surgical removal. Although the mechanism involved in cortisone-induced cataracts is not clear, cortisone drugs may dehydrate the lens or alter carbohydrate metabolism in the lens. Small posterior cataracts have been observed to resolve in some asthmatic children after they changed from oral prednisone to inhaled cortisone drugs.

The risk for cataract formation in younger people is negligible. Dr. Estelle Simons from Canada's University of Manitoba looked at the risk for cataracts in young children treated with inhaled cortisone and found no cortisone-induced cataracts in ninety-five people who underwent eye examinations. In summary, the risk for cataract formation is minimal for people taking low to moderate doses of inhaled cortisone drugs.

Psychiatric Side Effects

Psychiatric side effects to inhaled corticosteroids are rare, while such side effects to oral cortisone drugs are not uncommon. Frequent complaints include depression, irritability, and mood disturbances. The risk of psychiatric side effects is dose-dependent. Such side effects disappear once the oral cortisone is tapered or discontinued. Those people who require long-term oral corticosteroids and experience significant psychological side effects may benefit from antidepressive therapy.

Cortisone Withdrawal

When asthmatics previously dependent on oral cortisone taper or stop oral cortisone, they may experience many unpleasant side effects. Typical withdrawal symptoms include loss of energy, poor appetite, severe muscle aches, joint pains, and a flare-up of co-existing problems like arthritis, hay fever, or eczema that were masked by the oral cortisone. Sometimes the symptoms of cortisone withdrawal are so severe that the drug has to be tapered slowly over several weeks or months.

CHAPTER TWELVE

The Leukotriene Modifiers

In 1938, asthma scientists discovered a new class of chemical mediators called slow-reacting substance of anaphylaxis, abbreviated SRS-A.
Laboratory research over the next two decades found that SRS-A was
composed of several chemicals called the leukotriene (pronounced lu-
ko-try-een) mediators. High levels of leukotriene chemicals were found
in the sputum and urine of people with asthma, leading to speculation
that they might be important triggers of bronchial asthma. This discovery led to the development of several drugs that block the actions of
the leukotrienes. These drugs, known as anti-leukotriene drugs or the
leukotriene modifiers (LTMs), are the first new class of asthma drugs
to be introduced in twenty-five years.

LTMs have bronchodilating and anti-inflammatory activity. They
block bronchospasm induced by aspirin in aspirin-sensitive asthmatics.
Early clinical trials with the LTMs in mild to moderate asthma showed
improvement in symptom scores and a decreased need for beta-agonist
rescue drugs. When LTMs were compared to an inhaled cortisone
drug, the people on the inhaled cortisone drug had better lung functions, but there was little difference in symptom scores or beta-agonist

use. One study found that people on high doses of inhaled cortisone were able to cut their inhaled cortisone dose in half when an LTM was added to their treatment program. Thus, these drugs have a cortisone-sparing effect, which means that they can lower the daily dose of inhaled cortisone needed to control asthma. One distinct advantage of the LTMs is that they come in pill form. Most studies show that people are more compliant when asked to take a pill once a day as opposed to using an inhaler two to three times a day.

First-Line Therapy?

Should the LTMs be used as a first-line controller therapy or monotherapy (one drug only) in persistent asthma? This important question is the subject of an ongoing debate between asthma specialists. Dr. Jeffrey Drazen from Partners Asthma Center in Boston, Massachusetts, believes that the LTMs can be used in place of inhaled cortisone in mild persistent asthma. Drazen notes that these drugs are easier to take. They all come in pill form, and people do not need extensive education techniques on inhalers and spacer use. Other asthma experts, like Dr. Sally Wenzel from the National Jewish Asthma Center in Denver, Colorado, feel that LTMs should not take the place of the inhaled cortisone drugs that are the cornerstone or "gold standard" in the management of persistent asthma.

I tend to side with Dr. Wenzel on this issue. Inhaled cortisone drugs have a longer track record, and there are minimal risks for people taking conventional doses. More importantly, inhaled cortisone drugs have been shown to have a greater anti-inflammatory effect that may prevent remodeling or long-term lung damage. At the present time, the LTMs can make no such claim, as they have only been around for a few years.

Some studies have found that LTM-treated patients were more likely to need an emergency visit or hospitalization for asthma whereas

ICS patients had less inflammation in their lungs. One in every four people does not respond to an LTM.

Side Effects of the LTMs

The LTMs have been tested in thousands of people and have been found free of significant side effects. While headaches and rashes were the most common side effects, the incidence was no more common than in the placebo group. The first LTM modifier released in the U.S., zileuton (Zyflo), may alter liver metabolism, as one to two percent of people in clinical studies had elevated liver enzymes. Liver function studies are recommended in the first few months of therapy with Zyflo.

In December 2000, a report in the *Annals of Internal Medicine* described three middle-aged women who developed a severe liver injury while taking zafirlukast (Accolate). One of these women required a liver transplant. These cases prompted the manufacturer of Accolate to revise its drug package insert to indicate that severe hepatitis and liver failure may occur in people taking Accolate. It is estimated that more than 1 million people have been treated with Accolate, so these toxic liver reactions are very rare.

Another noteworthy adverse effect of the LTMs has been the rare development of an entity called the Churg-Strauss Syndrome, a syndrome characterized by vasculitis or inflammation of blood vessels throughout the entire body. The Churg-Strauss Syndrome usually occurs in people who have tapered or stopped taking an oral cortisone drug like prednisone after starting an LTM. It appears that the LTMs do not directly cause the Churg-Strauss Syndrome. The vasculitis is due to an unmasking of this syndrome when oral steroids are tapered or discontinued. Most of the people who develop the Churg-Strauss Syndrome have severe persistent asthma. The rate of this unusual complication appears to be very rare—about one in every twenty thousand treatment-years.

Summing Up

I feel LTMs can sometimes be used alone in cases of very mild persistent asthma—especially in children, or if exercise-induced asthma is a prominent feature, or when there is a strong steroid phobia on the part of the patient or family. One distinct advantage of LTMs is that oral administration may relieve nasal symptoms in hay fever and control hives in asthmatics with chronic urticaria. When there is a risk of permanent lung damage or remodeling in people with more persistent and severe asthma, LTMs are at best add-on drugs. Physicians should be aware that some LTMs are potentially liver-toxic, and people should be observed for signs and symptoms of hepatitis. Long-term experience with LTMs will ultimately lead to a better understanding of these drugs and define their proper place in asthma therapy.

CHAPTER THIRTEEN

Additional and Futuristic Asthma Drugs

Antihistamines in Asthma

Doctors have been traditionally taught to avoid using antihistamines in asthma because of their potential to dry up secretions and worsen asthma. Many antihistamines contain a warning on their label that states that they should not be used in asthma. This is an unnecessary precaution, as most asthmatics can safely take an antihistamine aggravating their asthma. People who do experience increased coughing or wheezing after taking an antihistamine should avoid them.

Previous efforts to treat asthma with older antihistamine drugs, like Benadryl, were unsuccessful because of their sedating tendency. Evidence now suggests that the new non-sedating antihistamines may play an expanded role in asthma. Today's newer drugs like Claritin, Allegra, and Zyrtec have been a godsend to people with allergic rhinitis or hay fever.

Expectorants and Asthma

One of the calling cards of asthma is an overproduction of thick mucus that is difficult to cough up or expectorate. Thus, you might think that expectorants or drugs that thin out mucus would be useful in asthma. Unfortunately, most expectorant drugs are relatively useless in asthma. While some of the newer expectorants may be of some help, the best (and cheapest) of all expectorants is plain water.

The Antibiotic TAO

Years ago, asthma researchers discovered that an erythromycin-like antibiotic, called troleandomycin or TAO, helped people with severe cortisone-dependent asthma. TAO interacts with cortisone by prolonging the half-life of cortisone in the body. This effect, which is known as the steroid-sparing effect, allowed cortisone-dependent patients to take less cortisone. Even though TAO reduces the total cortisone requirements, people still had significant cortisone side effects despite a lowering of their total cortisone dose. In effect, TAO doubles or triples the dose of oral cortisone. Two reports of a fatal varicella (chicken pox) infection in people taking TAO and the cortisone drug methylprednisolone (Medrol) have dampened my enthusiasm for TAO therapy.

Antibiotics in Asthma

I used to feel that most asthma doctors, including myself, were guilty of over-prescribing antibiotics in asthma relapses. While doctors know that most asthma relapses are triggered by viral, not bacterial, infections, it is difficult to withhold an antibiotic from a wheezing patient coughing up thick yellow-green-colored phlegm or sputum.

Vaccines in Asthma

You can prevent an asthma relapse caused by the influenza virus by taking an annual flu shot. Sometimes, the flu vaccine induces a mild asthma flare-up, but studies show it is worth the risk as immunized people have fewer flu-like illnesses and hospitalizations. I recommend flu vaccine for all my patients, including children, with persistent asthma. Even though bacterial infection is an infrequent cause of an asthma relapse, people with chronic asthma, especially those over fifty years of age, should receive the pneumonia vaccine. Children with persistent asthma should receive the new pediatric pneumonia vaccine.

Gold Therapy

The recognition that chronic inflammation plays a role in asthma suggests that drugs used to treat other inflammatory diseases, like rheumatoid arthritis, might be beneficial in asthma. Gold therapy has shown a favorable response in some people with severe asthma. The drawbacks to gold therapy are twofold. It may require four to six months before any benefit is seen, and responders are limited to people with allergic or IgE-mediated asthma. Side effects to gold therapy include skin rashes and stomatitis (inflammation of the mouth and tongue). Oral gold or Auronofin has been studied in America in a few oral cortisone-dependent people with favorable results. Additional studies are needed to confirm these findings.

Methotrexate Therapy

The safety and effectiveness of low doses of methotrexate, an older cancer drug, has been demonstrated in children and adults with rheumatoid arthritis. Seattle's Dr. Michael Mullarkey reported the potential value of methotrexate in severe asthma. Long-term studies by Mullarkey have shown that methotrexate can be administered over an eighteen- to twenty-eight-month period. Low-dose methotrexate may provide an alternative to the chronic use of high doses of daily or alternate-day prednisone. Two other methotrexate trials demonstrated improvement in asthma and a reduction in the need for oral prednisone. The most common side effects of methotrexate are gastritis, mouth irritation, and low blood counts.

An eighteen-patient, placebo-controlled study at the National Jewish Hospital in Denver, Colorado, suggests that more aggressive management of asthma is necessary before entering into a methotrexate program, as 40 percent of the people on the placebo drug in this study showed significant improvement. Methotrexate is an experimental asthma drug. You and your physician should be fully aware of the potential risks and benefits of methotrexate therapy, as there are no guidelines for its use in asthma.

Another cancer-type drug being looked at in severe asthma is cyclosporin A. This compound was studied in twelve people with severe cortisone-dependent asthma. Half of the cortisone-dependent patients were able to reduce their oral prednisone dose, from 30 milligrams a day to an average of 10 milligrams a day.

Experimental Asthma Drugs

Hydroxychloroquine is an antimalarial agent used in rheumatoid arthritis and systemic lupus. A study of hydroxychloroquine in patients with cortisone-dependent asthma found a reduction in the need for oral cortisone. Azathioprine is another antimetabolite shown to be a cortisone-sparing agent and immunosuppressant in a number of inflammatory diseases. In two studies in asthma, no benefit was seen with azathioprine. The popular anti-inflammatory gout medicine, colchicine, was administered to ten asthmatics, who showed small improvements in symptom score and less need for beta-agonists, but no change in lung functions.

Intravenous Gammaglobulin

Gammaglobulin, the major antibody of our immune system that protects us from many major infectious diseases, has been successfully used in immune deficiency disorders. Monthly intravenous infusions of gammaglobulin increase antibody levels and protect against many viral and bacterial infections. In higher doses, gammaglobulin acts as a modulator of the immune system by assisting the immune system in regulating the production of IgE antibody and the T-cells that cause chronic inflammation in asthma. Eight steroid-dependent asthmatics from the National Jewish Hospital, age eight to seventeen, received high-dose intravenous gammaglobulin for six months. They had a three-fold reduction in their need for oral cortisone and increased pulmonary function tests, but no change in bronchial hyperreactivity. The positive findings in this small study suggest larger trials are needed with gammaglobulin, particularly in view of the fact that intravenous gammaglobulin costs approximately $30,000 per year.

Lidocaine Therapy

Severe asthmatics who require oral cortisone are constantly being studied by asthma researchers in a never-ending search to determine why their asthma is so severe. Mayo Clinic doctors set out to analyze the mucus or sputum produced in the lung of people with severe asthma. In their study, an instrument called a bronchoscope was passed down into the lung, and mucus was collected for laboratory analysis. In order to minimize discomfort from the procedure, the windpipe or trachea was sprayed with a local anesthetic, lidocaine or Xylocaine—the same anesthetic drug used by your dentist during dental work.

Much to the surprise of the investigators, these cortisone-dependent asthmatics felt much better after the procedure. Several people were able to cut back on their daily dose of prednisone. As the only variable in this study was the use of nebulized lidocaine, the Mayo Clinic doctors set up a pilot study to look at the effects of spraying lidocaine into the lungs of oral cortisone-dependent asthmatics. The results were quite impressive. Many of the subjects tapered or discontinued their oral prednisone. They then studied six children with severe asthma. Five of the six children given lidocaine were able to discontinue their oral cortisone three months after starting lidocaine.

The one advantage of lidocaine over other experimental asthma drugs like gammaglobulin, cyclosporin, and methotrexate is its more favorable safety profile. These preliminary findings have spawned additional investigations on local anesthetics in the treatment of severe asthma. Again a word of caution! This type of experimental asthma therapy should only be done in specialized clinics or asthma centers experienced in treating severe cortisone-dependent asthma.

Magnesium Therapy

Magnesium, the fourth most abundant mineral in the body, is a trace mineral found in leafy green vegetables, nuts, peas, beans, and whole-grain cereals. Magnesium regulates a series of enzyme systems critical to cellular metabolism. The exact mechanism by which it exerts its effects is unknown.

The possibility that magnesium had bronchodilating properties was reported in 1938. One rather fascinating story on magnesium and asthma comes from the DMZ Rehabilitation Clinic located on the shores of the Dead Sea in Israel. The Dead Sea is a unique reservoir of minerals, and the content of its salt or brine is high in chlorides, bromides, and minerals like magnesium. Apparently, a microclimate is formed by high winds in this area that produce a mineral-rich haze that contains magnesium. It is believed that exposure to this microclimate is responsible for improvement in a variety of medical conditions. Researchers at this DMZ Clinic feel that people with psoriasis, hypertension, and asthma improve significantly when they are directly exposed to this climate. Such exposure includes topical application of the brine and mud from the Dead Sea.

In 1994, doctors at the DMZ Clinic observed that asthmatic patients attending the clinic for allergic skin diseases experienced less asthma and needed fewer asthma medications. This beneficial effect that was documented by breathing tests and symptom scores persisted for several months after their patients returned home. One possible explanation for their improvement was that they breathed air with a higher concentration of minerals, including magnesium. Ongoing research at this center and elsewhere may eventually shed more light on the role of magnesium therapy in asthma.

Anti-IgE Therapy

IgE antibody is the immune protein that predisposes us to develop allergic diseases. The newest asthma-allergy drug approved by the FDA is the IgE antibody-blocking drug, Xolair, released by the FDA in 2002. Scientists have theorized that if you could shut down IgE production, you might cure asthma and other allergic disorders. Just a few years ago, this concept seemed to be nothing more than a dream. Now, thanks to enormous strides in immunology research, this dream has become a reality.

Three major biotech drug companies, Novartis, Genentech, and Tanox, partnered to get FDA approval for Xolair. This anti-IgE drug ties up circulating IgE antibody and prevents IgE from attaching itself to the mast cell. Preliminary studies in human volunteers at research centers in San Francisco and Denver found that IgE levels were reduced by 99 percent after receiving anti-IgE antibody. That's the good news. The bad news is that when the study subjects stopped taking the drug, IgE levels bounced back up to or above pretreatment levels. This rebound reaction is somewhat disturbing, as it looks like the drug will have to be taken at regular intervals on an indefinite basis for it to be effective.

In one study, Xolair and placebo injections were administered to 289 patients with allergic rhinitis once or twice a month for four months. Xolair-treated patients unresponsive to other therapies experienced a 45 percent reduction in symptoms. No adverse reactions occurred in the treated group. Xolair is now recommended for moderate to severe asthmatics over twelve years of age whose asthma is not controlled with conventional therapy. It may also find a niche in people with severe allergic rhinitis. Another place for this novel drug may be in people with severe life-threatening food (especially peanut) allergy. However, it hasn't been approved.

Are there any potential drawbacks to this approach to the treatment of allergic disorders? Perhaps we are messing too much with

Mother Nature. Remember that IgE antibody once protected man from primitive parasitic diseases.

One of the consequences of aging is that our immune system gets weaker as we get older. An aging immune system makes us more susceptible to all kinds of chronic and often fatal diseases. However, this winding down of the immune system is beneficial to many sufferers of asthma and hay fever who become less allergic and less symptomatic with age. It may be the only benefit of aging that I can think of. Yet, in my experience, many elderly people do not always "outgrow" their hay fever or asthma, and they continue to have significant allergic symptoms well into their sixties and seventies. Over the past thirty years, I have been very impressed by the overall good health of these "allergy-suffering senior citizens." They often look much younger than their stated age and frequently have no other medical problems other than hay fever or mild asthma. This observation, strictly a personal one, is not supported by any scientific studies. I wonder if it is possible that IgE antibody may somehow protect some individuals from other non-allergic diseases by keeping their immune system in the high-speed lane. An overactive immune system may be fighting off other chronic diseases seen in the aging population, including cancer. One preliminary study found a lower incidence of lymphoma in individuals with higher IgE levels.

The other risk of shutting down the pro-allergic IgE-Th2 side of the immune system with an anti-IgE antibody is that you might push the immune system over to the non-allergic Th1 pathway. Excess stimulation of this Th1 pathway may lead to autoimmune diseases. This scenario has been observed in primates given more advanced forms of an IgE-suppressing antibody. Thus, before I fully endorse and prescribe a product that suppresses the allergic-IgE antibody, I would like to see studies showing that suppression of IgE antibody does not have any adverse effects on other parts of our protective immune system over the long term.

Asthma Drugs of the Future

New asthma drugs have been slow in coming. Compared to the ava-
lanche of new medications for heart disease, high blood pressure, gastrointestinal problems, and migraine headaches, only two new classes
of asthma drugs, the leukotriene modifiers and the blocking antibody,
Xolair, have been approved for asthma in the past two decades. A variety of unique asthma drugs are under study. As there are approximately 150 million people in this world with asthma, the economic
incentive for pharmaceutical companies to develop new asthma drugs
is unlimited. Unfortunately, progress is painfully slow, as it takes several
years and millions of dollars to bring a new drug to the marketplace.

Prior efforts to develop asthma drugs in the 1980s and 1990s focused on the endpoint of asthma-bronchial hyperreactivity and inflammation. Today, research is aimed at the beginning of the immune
response, finding ways to block the immune system from traveling
down the asthma-allergy highway or to interrupt the allergic march.
As I will discuss in chapter sixteen, dealing with immunotherapy, the
final cure for asthma and other allergic disorders may lie in administering genetically derived products or DNA vaccines to allergy-prone
infants and young children before they start to develop symptoms of
an allergic disease.

New asthma drugs in the pipeline include Pumactant (Britannia
Pharmaceuticals), a dry powder that works on the surface of the
bronchial tree to protect against allergens and irritants. Two new
Japanese asthma drugs, baynas and seratrodast (Bayer Yakuhin Ltd.),
will target the thrombaxin A2 protein. GlaxoSmithKline is developing
a drug called Airflo to inhibit an asthma-inducing phosphodiesterase.
Immunex is studying an interleukin blocker called Nuance (the mediators coming out of the T-cells are called interleukins). Many other
drugs in this class have entered early clinical trials. These drugs, called
interleukin blockers, are probably several years away from FDA approval. As there may be eighty or more mediators involved in asthma,

Dr. Peter Barnes thinks the next generation of asthma drugs will be one big anti-mediator pill that blocks several mediators. Perhaps the most promising of the new drugs will be the inhaled cortisone drug, ciclesonide (Aventis), which is delivered once a day in an inactive form and activated in the lung and has minimal systemic absorption.

Proceed with Caution

I prefer to take the yellow flag approach to all new drugs. In other words, proceed with caution! Remember, most new drugs are tested on only one hundred to one thousand people. More serious or rare side effects may not be seen until the drug has been used by thousands of people. In the past, the FDA has been soundly criticized for taking too long to approve new drugs. Now the FDA may be acting too quickly. In 2004, the FDA review time for a new drug was down to fourteen months, compared to thirty-four months in 1993. Paying a special FDA fee gets you a speedier process.

Since 1997, several new FDA-approved drugs have been removed from the market after they were found to cause serious injury and death. These drugs included the ulcer and reflux drug, Propulsid; the irritable bowel syndrome drug, Lotronex; and the diabetes drug, Rezulin. The cholesterol-lowering drug, Baycol, was taken by seven hundred thousand Americans before it was removed from the marketplace in 2001. Destruction of muscle cells resulted in kidney failure and thirty-one deaths in the United States and nine abroad. Baycol was the twelfth prescription drug to be removed since 1997. Remember that Seldane, one of the most popular antihistamines of all time, was available for several years and used by millions of people before it was recognized that when it was taken with certain antibiotics or antifungal drugs it could trigger a serious and sometimes fatal cardiac heart rhythm.

CHAPTER FOURTEEN

Alternative Asthma Therapy

The term alternative or complementary therapy refers to nontraditional medical treatments that have neither been approved nor proven to be effective in controlled studies by the established Western medical community.

Alternative or complementary products include, but are not limited to, phytopharmaceuticals (herbal agents), homeopathic remedies, nutraceuticals, and anthroposophics. There is no financial incentive to test or study these products, as new drug applications are not needed. The United States Diet Supplement and Health Education Act (DSHEA) does not require proof of safety or efficacy by the FDA. The only way the FDA can remove an alternative medicine or herbal remedy is to prove that it is unsafe. This is in contrast to the United Kingdom, Germany, and Canada, where alternative treatments are closely regulated by the government.

Over the past decade, the popularity of alternative therapy has grown immensely. It is estimated that 40 percent of allergy and 20 percent of asthma sufferers in the United States use some form of alternative medicine. Millions of American health-care consumers spend more than \$15 billion on natural herbal supplements and \$30 billion for providers of alternative health care. More people visit alternative medical practitioners than primary care physicians—600 million visits to alternative care providers versus 400 million visits with primary care physicians. Nearly two thousand herbal products gross more than \$20 billion a year.

When you look back on the history of pharmacological products in medicine, alternative drugs are not all that new. The asthma drug cromolyn (Intal) was derived from ammi visnaga, a Mediterranean plant used by Arabic physicians to treat intestinal colic one hundred years ago. Theophylline was extracted from tea leaves and coffee beans. The heart drug digitalis comes from the foxglove plant. Aspirin arose from the bark of the willow tree, and penicillin was discovered when a laboratory investigator accidentally found that penicillium-like molds were killing bacteria.Why is alternative therapy becoming more attractive? Alternative remedies offer a ray of hope for many people confused by complicated drug programs. People fear traditional medicine and its outcome, as conventional prescription drugs cause more than one hundred thousand American deaths each year. Dissatisfied people constantly surf the Web to consult herbalists and seek alternative therapies. Courses in alternate therapy are now offered in medical schools and teaching hospitals. Most physicians, including myself, have underestimated the potential benefits of alternative therapy. A United Kingdom study found that nearly six in every ten asthmatics were using alternative therapy, and the majority found it to be beneficial.

The U.S. Congress has responded to this explosion in alternative therapy by creating the Office of Alternative Medicine (OAM). In 1998, the NIH launched the National Center for Complementary and Alternative Therapy, which has a yearly budget of \$100 million. Alternative therapies being investigated by the NIH include herbal remedies, nutritional supplements, acupuncture, hypnotherapy, relaxation techniques, and chiropractic therapy. Ongoing clinical trials are evaluating the use of St. John's wort in depression, shark cartilage in lung cancer, and ginkgo in dementia. Of the twenty thousand herbal supplements in the world, several that are recommended for additional study include echinacea, feverfew, milk thistle, and valerian. Preliminary studies on alternative therapies for asthma have had mixed results. In one yoga study, the combination of yoga with cleansing techniques, vomiting, diarrhea, and nasal throat irrigations increased lung functions and exercise capacity after two years of therapy. The results with acupuncture are mixed. In eight of thirteen trials the benefit was quite small. In 1998, thirty-six children who underwent massage therapy had a better attitude toward their asthma. When hypnosis was combined with relaxation exercises, study patients used fewer asthma drugs and had more symptom-free days.

Herbalism

The development of modern-day herbal remedies is based on the philosophies and beliefs derived from ancient Greek, Roman, Arabic, and Chinese cultures. The basic components of herbal remedies are botanical products derived from natural plant life. Herbs are any part of a plant, including the leaf, flower, root, stem, fruit, or bark, used to make a medicine, fragrance, or food flavoring. Herbal medicines are touted as a safer and more natural approach to health care. Herbal supplements are packaged in teas, powders, tablets, liquids, and capsules. Proponents of herbal medicine believe herbs contain naturally occurring chemicals with potent biologic and immunological activity.

The traditional Chinese medicine branch of herbalism relies on maintaining a balance between two forces, the yin and the yang, and the five major elements of fire, earth, water, metal, and wood. Many Chinese asthma herbs are derived from ma huang, the herb extracted from the ephedra bush. Chinese physicians or healers have used ma huang for more than four thousand years to treat asthma. The study of ma huang led to the development of a Western drug called ephedrine, a major ingredient of early asthma medicines in the twentieth century. Other popular herbal remedies include ginkgo biloba, believed to improve memory and thinking ability. Ginkgo is the number-one herbal remedy used by older people. St. John's wort is widely used by people with mood disorders. Glucosamine and chondroitin sulfate are popular alternative treatments for joint pain and arthritis. Some of the more common medical conditions for which people turn to alternative therapies include low back pain, allergies, and asthma.

Commonly used herbs in asthma include atropa belladonna, or deadly nightshade, where the primary ingredient is atropine, the basic ingredient of asthma cigars and cigarettes. Licorice root is a favorite of Chinese practitioners who recommend it as a cough suppressant. Saikoku-to, a popular herbal remedy in Japan, reportedly allows some asthmatic patients to reduce their doses of oral cortisone by prolonging the action of cortisone. Tylorphorsa indica has been used in India to treat asthma and bronchitis. Another Indian herb touted as a possible bronchodilator is coleus forskohli.

Herbal research is in its infancy. Only five thousand of the world's five hundred thousand plants have been studied. While the majority of herbal papers are written in Chinese or Japanese, millions of Americans with allergies and asthma utilize these unproven products. The typical herbal user is a well-educated, middle-aged Caucasian with a higher income. In other words, baby boomers are into herbal medicine big time. Some of the more popular herbal preparations subjected to analysis include ma huang, Minor Blue Dragon, Chai Ge Jie Ji Wan, ginkgo biloba, ginseng, and licorice root. Other asthma studies include the use of tea made with black pepper and cinnamon, doses of carbovegetables (vegetable charcoal), Ipecacuanha (ipecac), and juice therapy with onion and parsley juice. Butterbar is another herb under study. Sixteen people on inhaled cortisone who took butterbar for one week had reduced inflammation in their lungs.

Perhaps the most exciting study in Chinese herbal medicine and asthma to date was performed in mice. Researchers at Johns Hopkins and the Mount Sinai School of Medicine in New York City have found that a Chinese herb (MSSM-002), which contains fourteen different herbal extracts, had significant anti-inflammatory and anti-asthmatic properties. Using a mouse-asthma model, the investigators found that MSSM-002 was comparable to a cortisone drug. While a mouse is not a man, this promising study implies that herbal preparations could have potent anti-inflammatory properties.

Herbal Side Effects

Presently there are no standards in the United States governing quality or strength of herbal products. The United States lags far behind many European countries where herbal products are classified as drugs. It has been suggested that the FDA classify herbal products as OTC medications. This would require manufacturers to provide proof of safety and effectiveness. There are several obstacles in the way of controlling herbal products.

Many herbs will never be investigated, as the cost of bringing a new product or drug to the marketplace approaches $500 million. Even if such a product were developed, it would not be protected by patent rights. The general public suffers under the misconception that all plant products are safe. Since they have a decided pharmacological action, you should only use herbal treatments under the care of a qualified naturopath or herbalist, to avoid the common side effects listed below.

- Many herbs contain alkaloids that can damage the liver.
- Ma huang causes insomnia, tremors, urinary retention, and irregular heartbeats.
- Lobeline may cause paralysis, coma, and death.
- Sweet root contains oil of calamus, a potent carcinogen.
- Mandrake when misused can be a poisonous narcotic.

- Chamomile tea cross-reacts with ragweed and can cause allergic reactions in ragweed-sensitive people.
- Overdoses of lobelia have been linked to respiratory paralysis, fainting episodes, and psychological problems.
- Sassafras, or "spring tonic," has been linked to cancer in lab animals.
- Echinacea may cause allergic reactions in people sensitive to flowers of the daisy family, and aggravate diseases like lupus, tuberculosis, and multiple sclerosis.
- St. John's wort affects the action of the clotting drug Warfarin and the AIDS drug Crixivan.
- Licorice and grapefruit juice can interfere with blood pressure, steroids, and cancer drugs.
- Valerian and kava kava interact with anesthetics during surgery.
- A higher risk of cancer has been reported with aloe, rhubarb (colon cancer), and capsaicin (gastric cancer).
- Ginkgo biloba may cause excessive bleeding during surgical procedures.
- Ma huang or ephedra can cause sudden death or strokes.

A disaster at a Belgian weight loss clinic involved the use of appetite suppressants and Chinese herbs. After the Belgian clinic made a switch to a toxic herb, nearly a hundred people suffered kidney failure and several people died. Fortunately, the FDA is becoming somewhat more proactive in regulating herbal products. They recently ordered an allergy-fighting compound called AllerRelief pulled off the shelves of health food stores. This herb contains the toxin aristolochic acid, the substance that triggered the outbreak of kidney problems and bladder cancer in the Belgian weight loss clinic. Ephedra was banned by the FDA in 2003.

Presently there are too many unanswered questions regarding the rate of absorption in the body, dosages, and contaminants of herbal products. All users of herbal products should buy reliable brands and monitor publications dealing with the potential side effects and drug interactions of herbal medicines. Reliable sources for such information include *Consumer Reports,* NIH publications, Medline, and *Prevention Magazine.* You and your health-care provider should report all significant adverse reactions to herbal products to the FDA at http://www.fda.gov/medwatch/report/consumer/consumer.htm

Summing Up

Many health-care providers have been too bewildered to learn much about alternative herbal products. There are nearly two thousand herbal products currently available in the United States. Much of the care in this area is self-experimentation, where people are more willing to rely on an unregulated herbal remedy than take an asthma drug. There is a growing need for educational efforts in the field of herbalism. Ask your doctor to help you make an informed choice.

A recent article in *Consumer Reports* noted that conventionally trained doctors were learning to be more sympathetic and less scornful. However, when one looks at the potential side effects of herbal products and assesses the fact that most studies of herbal remedies in asthma and allergic disorders are poorly controlled and done in only a few patients, at the present time I cannot endorse or recommend any herbal medicine as a form of alternative care in the treatment of asthma or allergic disorders.

For additional information and reading materials, I recommend Natural Medicines Comprehensive Database, 3120 W. March Lane, PO Box 8190, Stockton, CA 95208; Tel: 209-472-2244; Fax: 209-472-2249; www.NaturalDatabase.com; Galaxy.com lists the top ten places on the Internet for alternative health-care information.

Dietary and Vitamin Therapy

I used to believe that there was no solid data on dietary therapy and asthma. However, new data is emerging that may change my thoughts on this issue.

An Italian study that looked at the dietary habits of 5,257 Italian children found children who ate foods rich in antioxidants, like cooked vegetables and citrus fruit, had less asthma and wheezing than children whose diet consisted of foods containing animal fats, white bread, butter, and margarine.

Children, especially those exposed to tobacco smoke, whose diets contained antioxidants like beta carotene, vitamin C, and selenium, had less asthma. Two new fish oil studies are interesting. One found that elite athletes with EIB (exercise-induced bronchospasm) who took fish oil supplements for three weeks had less allergy and EIB. Another study found that pregnant mothers who took fish oil gave birth to children who had less egg allergy and eczema in their early years.

Additional studies are needed to look at the overall effects of maternal diet during pregnancy and in early infancy. Some researchers feel that exposure to antioxidants and omega-3 fatty acids in a developing fetus or newborn infant may reprogram the immune system to prevent the development of immune-mediated diseases like asthma. The antioxidant vitamins, such as vitamin A (beta carotene), vitamin C (ascorbic acid), vitamin E (alpha-tocopherol), and vitamin B6 (pyridoxine), are our first line of defense against tissue injury and theoretically might benefit asthma sufferers.

No specific studies have examined the role of vitamin A in asthma. One study in 77,866 nurses that examined vitamin E intake in adult-onset asthma found a 50 percent reduction in asthma in women with the highest vitamin E intake. A study utilizing a case-controlled design found that asthmatics had lower than average levels of vitamin B6. While there is no solid data to support the use of specific vitamins in asthma, taking a daily multivitamin can't hurt. Vitamin B6 is found in cereals, bread, whole grains, liver, spinach, bananas, fish, poultry, meats, nuts, potatoes, green leafy vegetables, and avocadoes.

The Pros and Cons of Acupuncture

Ancient Chinese acupuncture involves inserting fine needles into various points on the body to restore the balance of energy flow throughout the body. While acupuncture has been widely used in China for asthma, the rise in popularity of acupuncture therapy for asthma in Western societies is not supported by clinical studies. One extensive review of acupuncture in asthma concluded that any possible benefit was mild at best. Anyone contemplating acupuncture should be sure their acupuncturist is certified by the National Certification Commission for Acupuncture and Oriental Medicine. Serious side effects are rare when acupuncture is performed by trained, certified professionals.

Yoga

Exercise, meditation, and control of body functions have played important roles in medical practice and religion, especially in India. Breathing exercises and ritualistic chanting are often used as a means to aid meditative self-hypnotism, attain relaxation, and decrease energy use. Such techniques are thought to benefit asthma, perhaps by reducing airway reactivity. Meditation may also lower oxygen consumption. Tantric yoga is a combination of cosmic or religious meditation and slow deep breathing to improve the distribution of energy flow through the body. Such practices are alleged to provide serenity and reduce fatigue. The Chinese have developed many forms of ritualized exercise, both for individual and group practice. The most popular of these practices is tai chi, where slow rhythmic body movements are associated with deliberate breathing.

The Ancient Art of Homeopathy

Homeopathy is a two-hundred-year-old system of medicine in which diseases are treated with diluted extracts of biological or plant extracts. Homeopathy is the most popular form of alternative therapy in France, where it is used by more than one-third of the population.

Homeopathy is also increasing in popularity in Germany and the United Kingdom. In Britain, nearly one-third of general practitioners prescribe homeopathic remedies. The credibility of homeopathic medicine was given a boost by a report published in *Nature* in 1988. This paper from Paris demonstrated that homeopathic remedies lowered allergic or anti-IgE antibodies. A recent study randomized two groups of asthma sufferers. One group received an oral homeopathic preparation of a standard allergen and the other group received a placebo. All patients were allowed to take their usual medications. After four weeks, symptom scores, pulmonary function tests, and bronchial responses to histamine showed significant improvement in the treated group compared with the placebo. This is too small a study to hang your hat on, and additional data is needed before endorsing homeopathic therapy. The most recent study on homeopathy by Dr. Adrian White studied ninety-three children at the Peninsula Medical School in Exeter, England, and found no improvement in their asthma when homeopathic therapy was added to their usual asthma medications.

Chiropractic Manipulation

In 1895, Daniel David Palmer introduced chiropractic care by claiming that many diseases could be managed by spinal manipulation. Chiropractic care is now the third largest form of primary care in North America with 65,000 practitioners in the U.S. and 6,000 in Canada. Classic chiropractic theory states that vigorous manipulation readjusts the spinal column, removes nerve interference or spinal stress, and alleviates the symptoms of many chronic conditions including asthma. Current practice differs considerably from Palmer's original teachings. Chiropractic therapy has evolved into a holistic, non-drug-oriented form of care. Chiropractors often prescribe elaborate elimination diets with vitamin, mineral, and antioxidant supplements to complement their use of massage and manipulation. Colon cleansing, heat and cold therapy, and other approaches alleged to remove toxins from the body are also popular. Specific chiropractic spinal manipulative therapy for asthma was recently reported to be no more effective than sham manipulation. While there is no doubt that chiropractic therapy can help back pain, there is no evidence that spinal manipulation is of any benefit in asthma. In 1998, a study published in the *New England Journal of Medicine* compared active and simulated chiropractic manipulation in ninety-one children with active asthma. All children received four months of chiropractic treatment consisting of active or sham spinal manipulation. No difference in asthma symptoms or pulmonary functions was found in either group.

CHAPTER FIFTEEN

Environmental Controls

In my opinion, the most neglected area in asthma and allergy therapy is environmental control. When simple steps are taken to eliminate common irritants and allergens from one's environment, dramatic improvement and even clinical remission is a distinct possibility. Unlike medication programs, which are costly and may cause serious side effects, environmental controls can be put into place without risk, family disruption, or major medical expense.

Invasion of the Dust Mites

Numerous studies have proved the value of creating a dust-mite-free bedroom. In a classic British study, nine dust-mite-allergic asthmatics moved into a hospital room where they carried on with their normal daily activities and took their usual asthma medicines. After sleeping in the hospital room for a few nights, all nine subjects were less symptomatic, took fewer asthma medications, and showed improvement in their breathing tests. Dr. Andrew Murray studied two groups of children with allergic asthma in Vancouver, Canada. One group did not make any changes in their environment, while the second group instituted strict environmental dust mite controls. After one month, children who slept in the relatively dust-free bedrooms had far less wheezing and used fewer asthma medications than children who made no changes in their bedroom environment.

In temperate and subtropical climates there is a seasonal variation in dust mite levels, with some areas showing a substantial rise in mite populations in the autumn. In many areas this pattern of mite prolif-eration directly coincides with seasonal increases in asthma relapses and asthma hospitalizations. Dust-mite-allergic asthmatics should focus on their bedroom and family room—the two most frequently in-habited areas of the home. A typical child spends 80 percent of his or her in-home time in the bedroom. An adult who averages eight hours of sleep a night will spend one-third of their life in a bedroom envi-ronment. The ideal dust-mite-free bedroom should be simply fur-nished and easy to clean. You should focus on two areas—the bedding and the carpeting. Pillows, mattresses, box springs, and comforters should be enclosed in zippered airtight mite-proof covers. Avoid cheaper plastic covers, which are hot and sticky in the summer and cold and clammy in the winter. Comfortable, well-designed, durable, synthetic covers can be obtained from local department stores and al-lergy retail stores. Mail-order houses specializing in allergy-free prod-ucts usually have the best prices and quality product lines. New products are lightweight and feel like linen.

Down or feather pillows, a favorite breeding ground for mites, should be replaced with Dacron or polyester pillows and covered with a mite-proof encasement. The best blanket is a washable cotton or synthetic blanket. All bedding, including sheets, should be hot-cycled at 140 degrees Fahrenheit at least twice a month. Avoid electric blan-kets that keep the dust mites cozy and warm.

The most important factor in controlling dust mite growth is hu-midity. Keep home humidity levels under 50 percent with dehumidi-fiers or air conditioners. Super-tight homes should be well ventilated, and kitchen exhaust fans should be installed. Whenever possible, homes in warmer humid climates should utilize central air conditioning to reduce dust mite and mold growth. Additional steps include covering heating or air-conditioning vents with filters, keeping closet doors closed, and avoiding heavy drapes in the windows.

The second most mite-laden area of the home is in the rugs or carpets. The ideal bedroom or family room flooring is a wood or vinyl floor with washable area rugs. When carpeting cannot be replaced, commercial carpet cleaners or mite-killing chemicals, called acaricides, can be applied to the carpets once or twice a year. One acaricide, called Acarosan, has been marketed in the United States. Another effective anti-mite spray is Allergy Control Solution, sold by Allergy Control Products. You cannot remove mites from a carpet by compulsive vacuuming, as mites burrow deep into the carpet and hold on fast with the little sucking pads on the ends of their legs. Normal steam cleaning is likewise an ineffective way to kill mites. One new method that combines active heat and steam treatments by delivering hot air and steam to mattresses, carpets, and furniture reduced mite levels and bronchial hyperreactivity in asthmatic people. In summary, I believe covering bedding and carpet removal to be the two most important steps in dust mite environmental control. Carpets in schools and public buildings may be another area for exposure to dust mites and animal allergens.

Containing Cockroaches

Over the past three decades, asthma specialists have become aware that cockroaches play an important role in asthma. Cockroaches have been reported to trigger asthma in many parts of the world, including Southeast Asia, Central America, India, South Africa, and Europe.

Inner-city asthmatics have a much higher incidence of cockroach allergy. In some urban asthma clinics, one in every four asthmatics is allergic to cockroaches. There is also an increased risk for cockroach exposure in public buildings like supermarkets, grocery stores, restaurants, department stores, and movie theaters. A cockroach allergy skin test is available; but a positive cockroach test does not mean that you have cockroaches in your home. The skin test may remain positive years after exposure to cockroaches.

I have seen several patients with a positive skin test due to past exposure to urban apartments in their student days or when they lived in semitropical or tropical climates. When the cockroach test is positive and there is no history of prior exposure, I tell the patient or family they may have a cockroach problem and to call their local exterminator, as cockroach removal often requires vigorous extermination procedures.

Typical extermination measures include removing food sources, setting bait traps, and using insecticide sprays. Removing carpets from the bedroom may also be helpful.

The Lowdown on Mold

In many damper climates, it is virtually impossible to avoid outdoor molds. Many mold-allergic asthmatics do well in dry desert or high-altitude climates. When given a choice, I advise my mold-sensitive patients to vacation or retire in Arizona, not Florida. Mold likes it hot and sticky. Therefore, the key to indoor mold control is controlling temperature and humidity levels. Use a humidity gauge to monitor humidity levels throughout the home. Use air conditioners and dehumidifiers in homes where humidity levels are over 50 percent. Good ventilation with exhaust fans prevents mold buildup in books, bedding, kitchens, damp bathrooms, basements, and laundry rooms. Avoid carpeting in bedrooms and damp basements. Keep bathroom tubs, tiles, and shower curtains mold-free. Excess use of vaporizers or home humidifiers promotes mold growth within the home. Avid gardeners should avoid freshly cut grass, mulch piles, and raking leaves. Mold-inhibiting chemicals can be sprayed in areas where there is an excess buildup of molds, and mold-inhibiting paints can be applied to walls or ceilings.

Molds are also found in many foods. However, I feel the threat of mold reactions from foods is vastly overrated. Common foods that grow molds include cheese, particularly aged cheese; homemade wine; pickled foods; dried fruits; mushrooms; and leftover bread. If these foods induce asthma symptoms, they should be avoided.

Once you discover indoor mold growing in your home the following steps should be taken:

- Clean with a bleach or anti-mold solution.
- Repair leaky roofs and remove mold sources such as damp carpets and moldy shower curtains.
- Dry out damp areas with air conditioners, exhaust fans, and dehumidifiers.
- Avoid carpeting on slab foundations or damp basement floors.
- Live and play above ground. Whenever possible, mold- (and dust-mite) sensitive people should avoid sleeping in basement- or cellar-level family rooms or bedrooms.
- Ventilate damp rooms and crawl spaces under the house.
- HEPA air filters will help reduce the number of mold spores.

Stachybotrys Mold

Stachybotrys is a slow-growing black mold that flourishes on materials with high amounts of cellulose, like wood, dry walls, plaster board, and ceiling tiles. It will not grow on bathroom tiles, concrete, or food. What makes this mold especially dangerous is that it produces a toxin that can cause a fatal bleeding lung disorder in infants. An outbreak of Stachybotrys disease in Northern Ohio followed severe flooding in the spring of 1994. Dozens of cases were reported in infants, a few of whom died.

In 1998, the American Academy of Pediatrics issued a policy statement that severe water damage and mold growth pose a risk for infants, and they recommended prompt cleaning (within twenty-four hours) of any water damage inside a home. This policy statement recommended removing any saturated cardboard, dry wall, or paper products that could serve as a food source for the deadly Stachybotrys mold.

Animal Allergens

Note: Presently there is an ongoing debate as to whether pet exposure is a friend or a foe. The following section applies to those people who know they are allergic to household pets.

There is a strong companionship that develops between man and animals. Animals, like dogs, may be needed for security purposes. The emotional benefits of owning a pet may have to be weighed against their capability to induce asthma or allergic rhinitis. Dogs and cats are the most frequent offenders, but any furry or feathered animal, including gerbils, guinea pigs, hamsters, birds, rats, and rabbits, can trigger asthma. Once you become allergic to any one species of animal, you are quite likely to develop an allergy to other furry or feathered animals when given the proper exposure.

Many allergists insist on animal removal. When allergic animal owners are unwilling to give up their pets, a compromise may be necessary. Limited exposure may be an acceptable approach.

- Keep the animal outside the home or out of bedrooms.
- Routine grooming is essential.
- Treat a pet's skin conditions aggressively.
- Maintain wood floors and leather or vinyl furnishings.
- Wash your hands immediately after touching an animal.
- Reduce carpeted surfaces in the home by using hardwood or vinyl floors with washable scatter rugs.
- Use HEPA air purifiers.

Controlling Dog Allergen

Dog allergen behaves much like cat allergen in that it is easily airborne. Dog- and cat-allergic individuals begin to sneeze and wheeze immediately after entering a home where these animals reside.

There is some encouraging news for dog lovers and families unwilling to part with their dogs. In 1999, a study in England measured dog allergen levels in homes before and after dogs were washed and shampooed twice weekly. Significant reductions in airborne allergen and reduced amounts of allergen in the dog's clippings were found. No effect was noted when the dogs were vacuumed. This survey concluded that you should wash your dog at least twice a week, as allergen levels increased just three days after washing.

Another way to minimize exposure to dog allergen is to confine the dog and keep it out of the bedroom and family room. Factors that increase dander production or cause excess shedding of hair or skin should be controlled. Dogs with common skin conditions like fleas and seborrhea that lead to excess dander production and dry skin will require special attention from their owner or veterinarian. A non-allergic family member should perform routine grooming procedures outdoors, preferably. Commercial hypoallergenic cleansers and dog shampoos have not been shown to reduce allergen levels.

Controlling Cat Allergen

Cat allergy is more common than dog allergy, even though more homes house dogs than cats. This may be due to the fact that cat allergen is more widely dispersed in our society. Cat allergen is a very small, sticky, invisible particle that is carried about on the clothing of cat owners to all kinds of places, including churches, schools, and other public buildings.

Reducing cat allergen in a home where cats reside is a daunting task. It has been estimated that an average cat can carry 60 to 130 milligrams of cat allergen on its coat and can spread 100 milligrams of allergen on a carpet every day. This explains why you may not see any reduction in cat allergen levels months after a cat has been removed from a home if carpets are left in place. Therefore, whenever possible, carpet removal or extensive carpet cleaning is essential when a cat is removed from the home or a cat-allergic asthmatic moves into a dwelling previously occupied by a cat.

In contrast to mite allergens, HEPA (or high-efficiency particulate air) filters reduce levels of cat and dog allergen by 70 percent in rooms with polished flooring. In contrast, only a 30 percent reduction is achieved in carpeted rooms. Frequent vacuuming is somewhat helpful as long as the vacuum is equipped with a HEPA exhaust filter or double-thickness bag.

Controlling the source of cat allergen remains difficult. Cat allergen is produced in the salivary and sebaceous glands and is also found in the voided urine of cats. Studies from Johns Hopkins University Asthma Center and the University of Virginia have produced both good and bad news for cat lovers. The bad news is that when a cat is removed from the home, it may take weeks or several months to rid the home of cat allergen. Homes with carpeted floors accumulate cat allergen 100 times faster than homes with polished floors. The good news is that weekly washing of the cat with soap and water or plain water dramatically reduces levels of cat allergen in the home. Studies at the University of Virginia show that washing the cat on a weekly basis, removing carpets and upholstered furniture, using HEPA air purifying devices, vacuuming, and regular cleaning significantly lower cat allergen levels. Surprisingly, one recent study found that the color of cats might be important. People with dark-colored cats were two to four times more likely to have cat allergy symptoms.

One other common type of animal sensitivity is horse allergy. Avoidance is the easiest solution if you are allergic to horsehair, but this may be impossible for avid riders. Many horse-allergic people can tolerate exposure to horses if they take medications before riding and avoid barns and grooming procedures.

Controlling Pollen
While there are no surefire ways to completely avoid outdoor pollens, the following steps help reduce symptoms:

- Do not pick or sniff allergenic plants.
- Close home windows and use air conditioners.
- Use HEPA-type air filters in bedrooms or family rooms.
- Keep car windows closed during pollen seasons.
- Watch weather forecasts. Dry, warm, windy days promote high pollen counts, while rainy, colder days will lower the pollen load. Daily pollen counts in your area are available through the National Allergy Bureau at 1-800-9Pollen.
- If possible, plan outdoor activities later in the day, as pollen counts are higher in the early morning hours.
- When outdoors, wear a visor or cap and sunglasses to keep the pollen out of your eyes.
- Keep your lawn cut short, as longer, more mature grass generates more pollen.
- Shower and shampoo before going to sleep to keep pollen off your pillow and bed.
- If you live near a vacant lot that becomes a ragweed garden, cut the ragweed down in late July or early August before it pollinates. There is no need to cut down nearby pollinating trees, as tree pollen can travel many miles and such an action is not likely to reduce exposure to tree pollen.
- Do not dry clothes or bedding outdoors where it can collect pollen.

Home Humidifiers

Dry indoor air acts like a giant sponge, soaking up moisture from your respiratory tract and dehydrating your skin, mouth, nose, and lungs. Low humidity causes dry skin and nosebleeds, and it accelerates the transmission of respiratory infections between household members. The hazards posed by dry indoor air can be partially overcome by proper use of machines called humidifiers that add water vapor to the air.

Ideal in-home humidity, which varies with the local climate, is usually between 40 and 50 percent. An inexpensive instrument called a hygrometer can measure indoor humidity. When humidity levels fall below 40 percent during the heating season in the northern climates, it is time to use humidifiers in bedrooms or family rooms, especially in homes heated with fireplaces, coal, or wood stoves. To avoid mold buildup in the humidifier, frequent cleaning is a must. Rinsing with a bleach solution (one tablespoon per pint of water) usually does the trick. Do not add cleaning agents (other than bleach) or mold-inhibiting tablets to your humidifier, as they can produce toxic emissions. Overusing a humidifier during the non-heating season promotes mold and dust mite growth within the home. Humidifiers that directly attach to hot air heating systems are ideal breeding grounds for all kinds of organisms. Such units should be replaced, drained, or cleaned on a monthly basis. Ultrasonic cool mist humidifiers are safer and more efficient than the older cool-mist vaporizers and are less likely to grow molds.

Are All Air Purifiers Created Equal?

Some indoor allergens and air pollutants can be removed from your home or office with air purifier devices.

Air filters are classified by their efficiency, or ability to remove particles of various sizes. When you are filtering air, you want to remove the small, lung-damaging particles that are invisible to the naked eye. Most of the less expensive filters do not remove particles less than 10 microns in size. The best and most expensive filters are the HEPA, or high-efficiency particulate air filters. True HEPA filters are 99.97 percent effective at removing particles as small as three microns. This three-micron-sized particle is critical, as it is the particle size most likely to be inhaled deep into the lung.

The cost of HEPA filters varies depending on the size of the area or room where they are used. Smaller HEPA filters for a small eight-by-ten-foot bedroom cost around $100. Larger HEPA filters cost $300–$500.

The cost for a full HEPA system in a central air system is around several thousand dollars. Shop wisely—beware of less efficient filters not labeled as true HEPA filters. HEPA filters are very quiet and energy efficient, consuming no more electricity than a 40-watt bulb. Widely advertised portable table or desktop air purifiers are ineffective. Most medical insurance companies will not cover the cost of air purifiers. Studies have shown that air cleaners are not effective in controlling dust mites unless their use is combined with mite-proof mattress encasements. This observation is probably due to the fact that the larger-sized dust mite particles only become airborne when the surrounding air is disturbed. On the other hand, smaller-sized dog and cat allergens are more likely to be airborne and are easily captured by air cleaners. I advise pet-allergic asthmatics to install HEPA air purifiers in both their bedroom and family room.

Air Conditioners

The most useful appliance for people with mold or pollen allergy is a room or automobile air conditioner. Bedroom air conditioning protects the sleeping asthmatic during the early morning hours, when trees, grasses, and weeds begin to release their pollen. An air conditioner also indirectly lowers dust mite and mold counts by acting as a dehumidifier. Use an air conditioner that circulates indoor room air, as most air conditioners do not filter pollen from outdoor air. Air conditioners must be cleaned frequently to prevent buildup of dust, mold, and pollen. Automobile air conditioning is a must for any pollen-sensitive asthmatic who spends a lot of time traveling by car. People who do not sleep in an air-conditioned bedroom should install adjustable fiberglass filters in their bedroom windows.

Demystifying Dehumidifiers

Indoor relative humidity is the key factor determining the growth and survival of dust mites and molds within the home. A dehumidifier is just the opposite of a humidifier. It removes water vapor or moisture from the air, which in turn reduces the growth potential of molds and dust mites. In order to do this successfully, relative humidity must be maintained below 50 percent for at least twenty-two hours per day in areas where outdoor humidity levels are high. Dust mite populations usually peak in the summer months. Thus, removal of water vapor from the air is critical at this time of year. Dehumidifiers should be used in moist areas of the home, especially damp cellars or basements.

Beyond the Home

Day-care centers and schools are important sources of allergens. If your pet-allergic child has increased difficulty at the beginning of the school week or end of the school day, make sure that the student is not seated next to children who live with dogs or cats. Such children have been found to carry large amounts of animal allergens on their clothing. A simple change in seating may minimize allergen exposure. This principle obviously applies to adults who may be having the same difficulty in their workplace.

Summing Up

Proper environmental controls may cost several hundred dollars. This expense is justified, and more than offset by the savings in prescription drugs and medical care at the doctor's office or hospital. Although most medical health plans do not cover these costs, any expense directly related to improving your home environment, from buying mite-proof covers for your bedding to an expensive overhaul of your heating system, is a legitimate income tax medical deduction. Table 15.1 summarizes the ten basic steps in environmental control.

Traveling and Asthma

People with asthma should take special precautions when traveling. Avoid flying if you have a sinus or ear infection. Always carry a second

TABLE 15.1

TEN BASIC STEPS IN ENVIRONMENTAL CONTROL

1. Add dust-mite-proofing to the bedding.
2. Remove carpets from the bedroom.
3. Relocate, confine, or wash pets.
4. Do not allow smoking in the home.
5. Avoid strong odors and chemicals.
6. Install kitchen exhaust fans.
7. Use humidifiers with caution.
8. Use bedroom air conditioners.
9. Install HEPA air filters.
10. Install a dehumidifier in your damp cellar.

set of medications in your carry-on bag in case your luggage is lost or stolen. If you have to fly on a foreign airline that allows smoking, request a seat as far away from the smoking section as possible. Many airlines allow passengers to carry caged pets on board. The major airlines vary in their allowance for pets in airline cabins. American Airlines allows a maximum of five pets per cabin. Several other airlines limit the number of pets to one or two per cabin. Southwest Airlines prohibits pets completely. The animals have to be small enough to fit into a carrier that goes under the seat in front of you. This makes it quite likely that the caged pet is a cat as most dogs are too big to fit into the carrying device. If you are allergic to pets and encounter this situation, ask the flight attendant to change your seat. Pet-allergic asthmatics should contact their airline in advance and carry their medications, including a battery-powered nebulizer, to deal with an allergy or asthma attack.

Try to take an early flight and sit in the front of the plane or in a window seat where the air is fresher. There are anecdotal reports that passengers in first or business class get more fresh air as there are fewer passengers sharing the same space. One common problem for air travelers with asthma is dehydration resulting from exposure to the dry, poorly humidified air in aircraft cabins. Use a salt-water nasal spray and drink plenty of liquids to avoid dehydration. Avoid consumption of alcohol or caffeinated beverages that promote dehydration. Dry airline cabin air also promotes the dissemination of respiratory infections. Wash your hands frequently; it's the best way to reduce your chances of picking up a cold or viral infection from fellow passengers.

Peanut- and tree-nut-sensitive asthmatics are at risk when they fly, as small particles of aerosolized peanuts or tree nuts can trigger a severe allergic reaction (anaphylaxis) or an asthma attack. Peanut particles are released into the air when a bag of peanuts is opened. High levels of airborne peanut allergen occur when a hundred or more people on an airplane open bags of peanuts at the same time. Peanut protein has even been found in the filtering devices onboard commercial aircraft. There are reports of fatalities in airplanes at high altitudes in peanut-allergic fliers. In response to this risk, many commercial airlines no longer serve peanut snacks. Many carriers will exclude peanuts from a flight when so requested well in advance of the flight.

Hotels and motels are notoriously bad environments for dust-mite and mold-sensitive asthmatics. Carry your own pillowcase covers. Ask if your hotel offers a dust-mite-free or so-called "green room" with mite-proof bedding and air purifiers. Avoid sleeping in musty rooms with antiquated air conditioners or stuffed furniture. If you are mold-sensitive, request a room in a dry, sunny area away from indoor swimming pools. Avoid rustic cabins that have been shut up for long periods. Ask the owner to air out the cabin hours before arrival. Camping equipment also provides an ideal site for dust mite and mold infestation. Air out tents and sleeping bags before camping trips. Allow damp camping equipment to dry out before repacking.

When traveling by car, bus, or train, be on the lookout for potential irritants like dust mites, mold, pollens, perfumes, and air pollutants.

If possible, travel in the early morning when traffic is lighter and air pollutant levels are lower. Asthmatics should carry a portable nebulizer that is battery powered, or one that can be plugged into the car cigarette lighter. Before entering a car, turn on the air conditioner to clear out pollen or mold spores.

In some remote areas or foreign countries, you may be the "best asthma doctor" around. When traveling overseas for prolonged periods or on a frequent basis, consider joining organizations designed to help travelers with medical needs. The International Association for Medical Assistance to Travelers (IAMIT) is a nonprofit organization that provides a physician directory of English-speaking physicians who have trained in a Western country. IAMIT also provides a Traveler Clinic Record for your doctor to complete prior to travel. While there is no charge for an IAMIT membership, a donation is appreciated. For information, call 716-754-4883 or visit their Web site at www.sentex.net/iamit

The Travelers Emergency Network (TEN) offers members twenty-four-hour access to a worldwide network of physicians and provides contact information for doctors where you are traveling. The annual membership fee is $99. For information call 1-800-ASK-4TEN or visit their Web site at www.tenweb.com

Is Animal Exposure Protective?

To me, one of the more startling developments in the field of allergy and asthma in the past few years has been reports that exposure to pets may protect against asthma and other allergic disorders. Such reports triggered many studies that are both complex and confusing—even to allergy specialists like myself. It all started when Scandinavian researchers found children raised in homes with cats were less likely to be cat allergic or develop asthma. A Tucson, Arizona, study that tracked 1,246 babies since 1980 also suggested that early exposure to cats and dogs may be protective and pet avoidance in early life may not be useful. Dog exposure was found to protect against asthma in families with no history of asthma. A *JAMA* study looked at 474 children and found the presence of pets was protective. In fact, the more the better as it took two or more pets to see a drop in the rate of allergies and asthma. This animal exposure may also prevent the development of other allergies, like mold or grass allergy. The effect was more pronounced in boys than girls. Dogs may be the most protective. Surveys of children in Sweden and Wisconsin found that dogs lowered the risk while cats actually increased it.

There may be two distinct groups of infants and young children. One group develops asthma or allergy when exposed to animal allergens. The other group is protected by exposure to high levels of animal allergen and such protection may be permanent. One study found that IgG antibody levels to cats were highest in the group with the highest exposures. At the present time, there is no accurate way to pick out those infants and young children who will be protected by animal allergen exposure. More studies are needed to unravel this issue.

In summary, I now recommend that infants and children at risk for asthma and allergic disorders (defined by a positive family history of asthma and allergic diseases—especially in the mother) avoid exposure to household pets. I no longer tell non-allergic families who wish to prevent allergies in their children to rid their home of pets. Such families have no reason to give up household pets when expecting a new arrival. On the other hand, I advise against introducing pets into the home to prevent asthma or other allergic diseases. However, all these studies raise the intriguing possibility that early exposure to allergens, like cat allergen, either through allergy injections or natural exposure, may induce an immune response that signals the all-important T-cells and B-cells to produce mediators and protective antibodies that could prevent asthma and allergic diseases for a lifetime.

CHAPTER SIXTEEN

Immunotherapy in Asthma

In 1911, two pioneers in allergy research, Doctors L. Noon and J. Freeman, discovered that hay fever victims who were injected with an extract of grass pollen before the grass pollen season suffered fewer symptoms once the grass pollinated in early summer. Modern research has documented their astute observations, and allergy injections, or immunotherapy, is now an accepted treatment for many allergic conditions, including asthma, allergic rhinitis, and stinging insect allergy.

In immunotherapy, a dilute dose of an allergen is injected once or twice a week for three to four months. Each succeeding dose delivers a higher concentration of the allergen. These weekly injections build up to a maintenance dose that is usually the highest dose the patient can tolerate without risking an allergic reaction. Once this maintenance dose is reached, injections are given every two to four weeks and continued for at least three to five years year-round.

When allergy injections are deemed to be successful, they are continued for three to five years. When it is clear that allergy injections are not helping or are causing adverse reactions, they should be discontinued. People who are relatively symptom-free for two consecutive years or pollen seasons deserve a trial vacation from allergy shots. Highly allergic individuals or those with continued allergen exposure often require more than five years of allergy injections.

How Do Allergy Injections Work?

Allergy injections work by directly stimulating your immune system. When an antigen or allergen is injected into your body, the immune system handles this allergen in two ways. The T-cells release chemical mediators that signal the immune system's B-cells to stop making allergic or IgE antibody to the injected substance. The T-cells also stimulate the B-cells to produce a gammaglobulin or IgG antibody called a blocking antibody. Later on, when an allergen is confronted by the blocking antibody, it neutralizes or blocks the allergen before it can get to the mast cell and trigger an allergic antigen-antibody reaction.

The net result of all this immune interplay is a lower level of IgE antibodies, a higher level of blocking antibodies, and a decreased capacity to mount an allergic reaction. In essence, allergy injections may push the immune system in the direction of the non-allergic Th1 pathway and away from the Th2 allergy response. When allergy shots are successful, people have fewer symptom days and require less medication to control their hay fever or asthma.

Immunotherapy has not always been a well-accepted mode of asthma therapy. There are several reasons why doctors have questioned the value of immunotherapy in asthma. First, immunotherapy for asthma is a difficult treatment to study. There are relatively few well-designed, double-blind, placebo-controlled studies dealing with immunotherapy and asthma. In a double-blind study, some people get an active drug (in this case an injection with the actual allergen), while others receive a placebo or inactive drug. Neither the patient nor the doctor knows who is getting what until the study ends. Few people are willing to take the chance of receiving placebo injections (salt water) for several years.

The second reason for the poor acceptance of allergy shots in asthma is that many people with asthma do not have allergies. Scores of unscrupulous "shot doctors" fail to prescribe correct medications or implement proper environmental controls before they sentence their patients to years of worthless allergy injections. Such poor and inappropriate treatment has given immunotherapy a bad reputation.

In my earlier teaching days, I believed that allergy shots were effective in asthma when administered to carefully selected patients, but at that time there was no concrete proof to present to skeptical medical students or house staff. Fortunately, advances and discoveries in the field of immunology, combined with well-designed clinical studies, have conclusively shown immunotherapy to be effective in hay fever, stinging insect allergy, and allergic asthma. Immunotherapy with dust mites, pollens, and cat allergen significantly lowers the overall reactivity of the asthmatic lung. Immunotherapy reduces both the early- and late-phase response and skin reactivity to allergens. One proponent of immunotherapy, Dr. Jean Bousquet from Montpellier, France, notes that despite the best efforts in environmental control and optimal medical management, the rate of symptom control may only approach 50 percent. Bousquet has published several papers showing that immunotherapy is effective with dust mites and pollen allergens. Unlike many American allergists, Bousquet stresses the need to use single allergens; that means that each allergen is injected separately and not mixed together as one shot. This approach allows one to administer more precise doses of each allergen. Bousquet adds that the safety of immunotherapy has vastly improved with the availability of standardized allergy extracts.

One review of sixty-two immunotherapy studies published between 1966 and 1998 found that immunotherapy significantly reduced asthma symptoms, medication requirements, and bronchial reactivity. Another review of twenty well-controlled studies concluded that immunotherapy consistently improved asthma symptoms, reduced airway reactivity, improved pulmonary function tests, and lowered the need for asthma medications. This review suggested that immunotherapy is cost effective because it reduces the need for expensive asthma medications, emergency care, and hospitalizations.

Recently, an exciting study on grass immunotherapy in England found that low symptom scores continued for several years after immunotherapy was stopped. A report from Sweden and Denmark is of special interest to cat lovers. Dr. Gunilla Hedlin investigated the effects of three years of placebo-controlled cat and dust-mite immunotherapy in twenty-nine children with moderate asthma. Hedlin found a general reduction in asthma symptoms and bronchial reactivity after three years of treatment. Hedlin also noted an improvement in the tolerance to cat allergen exposure. This study is important due to the increasing prevalence of cats in our society. A Swedish study found that 53 percent of asthmatic schoolchildren were cat allergic. As cats are so abundant and cat allergen can be found anywhere, cat allergen immunotherapy may be the only way to control cat-induced asthma in some people.

Indications for Immunotherapy

Who needs immunotherapy? I generally use the following guidelines to determine when immunotherapy is indicated:

- Presence of allergic or IgE-mediated asthma for more than two years
- Excess loss of school and work days or repeated hospital visits
- Allergic asthma that is not responding well to medications or environmental controls
- Inability to tolerate asthma medications
- Coexisting diseases, such as allergic rhinitis or eczema
- Positive skin tests that correlate well with the clinical history
- Persistent asthma and exposure to cats in the home

Risks of Allergy Injections

Allergy injections are not entirely risk-free. They should always be given under the supervision of a physician. After receiving your injections, you should remain in the clinic or doctor's office for thirty minutes, as most injection reactions occur within this time frame. Allergy injections should not be self-administered at home or by well-meaning relatives, neighborhood nurses, or others who lack experience in administering allergy shots or treating systemic reactions induced by allergy injections. The most common injection reaction is a local swelling at the site of the injection. The size and intensity of this local reaction often determines the strength of the next dose. Sometimes you might experience what is called a systemic reaction, which means that you develop symptoms of an acute allergic reaction.

Mild systemic reactions cause itching and sneezing, while more severe reactions may induce asthma symptoms. Most injection reactions respond promptly to an antihistamine like Benadryl or an injection of epinephrine. Whenever a patient experiences a significant reaction to an allergy shot, the doctor should make a careful dosing adjustment prior to the next injection visit to prevent a recurrence of the systemic reaction.

In rare instances, a severe anaphylactic or allergic reaction may occur, blocking a patient's airway or causing a drop in blood pressure. Deaths from allergy injections and skin testing have been reported. Fortunately, they are extremely rare. Dr. Richard Lockey compiled data on forty-six fatalities associated with skin testing or allergy injections. These deaths took place between 1954 and 1985—a rate of about one a year. Persons at risk included those experiencing seasonal symptoms and people on beta-blocking drugs. Additional data in Lockey's study suggest that people at the greatest risk are women with unstable, severe asthma and low lung function tests. Our practice has stopped giving injections to people who fit this profile. In my opinion, allergy shots usually do not work very well in this particular group.

Treatment Failures

As with any form of medical treatment, immunotherapy treatment failures are bound to occur. The five most common causes of treatment failures in immunotherapy are the following:

- Allergy "shot doctors" treating people with non-allergic asthma
- Poor control of the environment, such as keeping pets in the home
- Failure to follow a regular injection schedule
- Development of new allergies not covered by the present injection program
- Inability to give an effective dose because of severe sensitivity to the injected allergen

New Frontiers in Immunotherapy

Over the past two decades I have been quite conservative, perhaps too conservative, in my approach to immunotherapy. When confronted with allergic patients, especially young children with developing allergies and allergic rhinitis or asthma, I usually relied on medications and environmental controls before starting allergy injections. In my experience, younger atopic children first become sensitized to tree pollen. These youngsters come into the office in April or May with severe nasal and eye allergies and wheezing. As the peak period for tree pollen levels in greater Boston occurs in early to mid-May, allergy specialists often call this "Mother's Day Asthma." When I treated typical pre-school children with tree pollen allergy, I held off recommending allergy injections until later childhood as many of these children would develop additional allergies over the next several years. Once these children developed a full-blown spectrum of allergies and were still having symptoms later on in childhood, I would recommend immunotherapy. I told these patients and parents that it took a long time—several months to a year or two—before immunotherapy took effect. There are several evolving reasons why this may be the wrong approach to immunotherapy.

Asthma and allergy drug therapy is aimed at reducing symptoms—the end result of the immune reaction that triggers the sneeze, wheeze, and itch response. Environmental controls attempt to prevent the immune reaction by removing the offending allergens. Neither of these treatments alters the basic cause of the asthma-allergy immune response. Only immunotherapy regulates the inflammatory response of the immune system.

Thanks to advances in immunology research, we know there are four effects from immunotherapy: an early effect, a persisting effect, a long-term effect, and a preventive effect. The early effect may be seen as early as eight to twelve weeks after starting allergy injections. The persisting effect is achieved during the next three to five years of therapy. New data has revealed that a long-term and preventive effect may last up to six years and perhaps indefinitely after stopping immunotherapy. Emerging evidence implies that there is a strong link between hay fever and asthma, as nasal allergies often precede the onset of asthma. It may all be part of one evolving disease process.

Fascinating studies by Dr. Bousquet have shown that administration of dust-mite immunotherapy to young children prevented the development of new allergies later on in childhood. This observation supports a theory by Dr. Thomas Platts-Mills that early natural exposure to an allergen (like cat allergen) may induce a state of immune tolerance and prevent allergy and asthma for a lifetime. French investigators are now starting pre-school children on allergy injections, which is an uncommon practice in the United States. Most American allergists wait until later on in childhood before recommending immunotherapy, as I do. An ongoing study in six European allergy centers, called the PAT or Preventative Allergy Treatment Study, found that non-asthmatic children with nasal and eye allergy who were started on immunotherapy to birch and grass pollen had a lowered incidence of asthma five years later than did allergic children who did not receive allergy injections.

These ongoing trials in Europe will determine if early administration of immunotherapy to young people with allergic rhinitis prevents the onset of asthma. I am very tempted to jump on this early-immunotherapy bandwagon. If these studies confirm that the early use of immunotherapy prevents the onset of additional allergies and asthma later on in childhood, I will radically change my indications for recommending allergy injections in children.

Allergy specialists have relied on natural products for the diagnosis and treatment of allergic diseases for a hundred years. One of the reasons for my conservative approach to immunotherapy was that many allergy extracts were not well-standardized and varied in quality and potency. While the quality and purity of allergy extracts have vastly improved over the past twenty years, the development of natural allergy extracts may have peaked. Tremendous progress in molecular biology now allows researchers to develop "super allergens" that will be more immunogenic and less allergenic. The use of the anti-IgE drug, Xolair, combined with immunotherapy injections, may also improve the results of immunotherapy. Traditional immunotherapy requires that the allergen be injected on a regular basis for several years. New allergens may be administered by mouth or inhaled into the nose or lungs. In March 2003, Italian researchers reported that oral or sublingual immunotherapy provided a long-lasting (four to five years) effect in sixty children with allergic rhinitis and asthma.

One very promising approach to immunotherapy is the development of antigens derived from proteins, called peptides. A peptide is actually a small fragment of a whole allergen that is altered by gene vaccination. Peptides directly affect the T-cells or lymphocytes that program the allergic-inflammatory reaction. Their advantage is that peptides have little risk of causing systemic reactions and can be given in higher doses. The development of other types of new allergens offers exciting prospects for allergen-specific therapy.

Another breakthrough will be the development of antigen-selective DNA vaccines capable of triggering a powerful protective immune response. One DNA-derived peanut vaccine has been shown to block sensitization and severe allergic reactions or anaphylaxis in peanut-allergic mice. Such therapy holds great promise for those people prone to severe life-threatening reactions to peanuts or tree nuts. Human clinical trials with such a product are now underway. Someday it may be possible to use a single allergen as a vaccination in infancy or early childhood and thereby prevent the development of asthma or allergy for a lifetime. These are only some of the possibilities that make immunotherapy the potential asthma therapy of the future.

CHAPTER SEVENTEEN

Special Types of Asthma

Cough-Variant Asthma

Coughing, wheezing, shortness of breath, and chest tightness are the major symptoms of asthma. Yet not everyone with asthma has all these telltale symptoms. In some people the only asthma symptom is a persistent cough. This form of asthma is called hidden or cough-variant asthma. Although cough has been recognized as a clinical feature of asthma for centuries, the recognition that cough may be the only asthma symptom was not appreciated until 1975, when Dr. Regis McFadden described a group of adult asthmatics whose only complaint was a chronic cough.

In 1982, I described a group of twenty-six children with cough-variant asthma. On long-term follow-up, three-fourths of these children with cough-variant asthma eventually developed more obvious signs of asthma. A recent review from Japan found that 30 percent of people with cough-variant asthma eventually developed typical asthma. Thus, cough-variant asthma may represent the early stages of persistent asthma. Dr. Peter Konig found that people with hidden asthma were often misdiagnosed and mistreated. Doctors failed to consider asthma as a possibility because the cough was not accompanied by wheezing, and they prescribed all sorts of ineffective medications, such as antihistamines, cough medicines, decongestants, and antibiotics. This is most unfortunate, as people with hidden asthma have a mild form of asthma that usually responds quite nicely to asthma medications.

The quality of a cough may help determine the cause of a cough. The cough due to a postnasal drip or a chronic sinus problem is usually a dry, nonproductive "tickle in the back of the throat" cough. The cough in tracheobronchitis or childhood croup is a barking-type cough. A goose-like honk or seal-like cough suggests a tic or habit-type cough. The cough from gastroesophageal reflux disease (GERD) is often worse at night or after eating, and is aggravated by stooping, reclining, or lifting.

The cough in hidden asthma is quite different. This cough has a bronchial quality, interrupts sleep, and is frequently triggered by cold air or exercise. The cough is often nonproductive (no mucus or sputum) and may persist for several years before the diagnosis of asthma is made. Risk factors that trigger cough-variant asthma include indoor and outdoor air pollution, tobacco smoking, domestic pets, and respiratory infections. In summary, a cough is a very common symptom among adults and children, as up to 30 percent of the general population have recurrent episodes of coughing that prompt a visit to the doctor's office. Medical studies have shown that 30 to 50 percent of people with a chronic cough may have unrecognized asthma. The take-home lesson here is an obvious one. Not all asthmatics wheeze, and if you, or someone you know, repeatedly coughs during sleep or exercise, cough-variant asthma is a distinct possibility. One way savvy parents, teachers, coaches, and gym instructors can uncover cough-variant asthma in children is to recommend an asthma evaluation for kids who repeatedly cough during sports, gymnastics, or exercise.

Nocturnal Asthma

Nighttime or early morning asthma, commonly called nocturnal asthma, was first described by Sir John Floyer. In 1698, Floyer wrote, "I have often observed the Fit always to happen after Sleep in the Night when Nerves are filled with windy Spirits and Heat of the Bed has rarefied the spirits and Humours." Nearly 90 percent of asthmatics wake up coughing or wheezing sometime during the night—most commonly between 3:00 and 5:00 a.m. Many people are unable to return to sleep using their rescue inhaler. Nocturnal asthma in children obviously affects all members of the household. The major consequence of nocturnal asthma is sleep loss that results in deterioration of daytime performance at school or at work. Dr. Margaret Turner-Warwick, from Brompton Hospital in London, England, collected data on more than seven thousand asthma sufferers who reported nocturnal wheezing. Sixty-four percent of these patients wheezed three out of seven nights a week, and more than one-third wheezed every night. The surprising finding of Turner's study was that nearly 25 percent of subjects who considered their asthma to be mild wheezed every night, and nearly half were awakened three times a week. Dr. Turner-Warwick concluded that being awakened at night by asthma symptoms was very common, and patients frequently overlooked nocturnal asthma.

Your health-care provider should instruct you to use peak expiratory flow meters to record the severity of your nighttime asthma and your response to treatment. People whose peak flow readings drop in the morning, called "morning dippers," are more prone to nocturnal asthma. Additional studies have found that nocturnal asthma attacks are more severe than episodes in the evening or early morning hours. Nocturnal asthma attacks are far more dangerous than daytime episodes, as most near-fatal and fatal asthma attacks occur suddenly and unexpectedly between midnight and 8:00 a.m.

The causes of nocturnal asthma are not fully understood. Some plausible explanations include a fall in circulating cortisone and epinephrine hormone levels, gastric reflux (regurgitating food or acid from the stomach), high allergen exposure to animal dander or dust mites in the bedroom, and nighttime changes in the tone of the nervous system's control of the airway. Recent studies found airway inflammation to be more severe in the prone versus the upright position, suggesting that the recumbency may be the main trigger of nocturnal asthma. It is quite likely that some or possibly all of these factors lead to an increase in airway reactivity severe enough to awaken a sleeping patient.

What is the best drug for the control of nocturnal asthma? First, anyone who awakens more than two to three times a month should take an inhaled anti-inflammatory or asthma-controlling drug daily. When this approach does not relieve nocturnal asthma, your healthcare provider has several options, including the addition of a long-acting beta-agonist, a leukotriene modifier, or a theophylline drug. I now prefer a long-acting beta-agonist drug such as salmeterol (Serevent) in nocturnal asthma. People who take a long-acting beta-agonist drug must be warned that the medication should not be used to relieve an acute attack of asthma and must never be taken without an inhaled cortisone drug. If one wakes up wheezing in the middle of the night, one should only use a short-acting bronchodilator like albuterol. When nighttime asthma does not respond to an inhaled cortisone drug, a long-acting bronchodilator, or a leukotriene modifier, I will prescribe a long-acting theophylline drug. I used to use theophylline drugs in all my patients with persistent nocturnal asthma, as studies from the 1970s and 1980s clearly showed that, at that time, theophylline was the best drug for nighttime asthma. However, many people cannot tolerate a bedtime dose of theophylline due its insomnia-inducing caffeine-like side effect.

Sometimes, changing the timing of the daily dose of asthma medications by taking your drugs later in the day—about 3:00 to 4:00 p.m.—successfully blocks nocturnal asthma.

Aspirin-Sensitive Asthma

First manufactured in Germany in 1899, aspirin remains the most widely used drug in the world. American drug firms produce nearly twenty tons of aspirin each year, and the American public consumes about 150 to 200 million aspirin tablets a day. For most of these millions of consumers, aspirin is a safe and effective drug. Not so for people with asthma, especially adults with asthma, who are ten times more likely to develop an allergic reaction to aspirin. A small group of asthmatics react adversely to aspirin and any drug that acts like aspirin. Symptoms of aspirin sensitivity include nasal congestion, hives, swelling, and wheezing. Asthmatics who react to aspirin are classified as aspirin-sensitive or aspirin-intolerant. Aspirin allergy is more common in people with chronic rhinitis, sinusitis, and nasal polyps. People are identified as being aspirin-sensitive only after they have experienced hives, swelling, or wheezing following ingestion of aspirin or other non-steroidal anti-inflammatory drugs (NSAIDs). Common NSAID medications that act like aspirin include ibuprofen (Advil or Motrin) and naproxen (Aleve, Naprosyn, or Anaprox).

Aspirin-sensitive asthma usually starts in adulthood and does not favor either sex or any ethnic group. After having been in good health, or having hay fever or mild asthma during childhood, the typical patient with aspirin-sensitive asthma experiences a cold or bronchial infection that does not resolve in ten to fourteen days. Nasal congestion and discharge persists for weeks. This is not your typical runny nose—it produces copious amounts of watery nasal discharge that require several handkerchiefs a day. These patients eventually lose their sense of smell or taste and develop grape-like growths in the nose called nasal polyps. Eventually, they develop asthma or experience an asthma attack after taking aspirin.

This triple-threat combination of sinus disease—nasal polyps, asthma, and aspirin allergy—is known as aspirin-sensitive asthma or Samter's Syndrome. This syndrome is named after Dr. Max Samter, who first described this condition. I might mention that I had the opportunity to train under this wonderful physician at his Asthma Institute in Chicago. A newer name for this condition is Aspirin Exacerbated Respiratory Disease (AERD), as it affects both the upper and lower airway. While aspirin asthma is rare in children, it is estimated that two million adults have AERD.

People with nasal polyps and asthma should not wait to have a reaction to aspirin before taking steps to avoid aspirin or NSAID medications. The only effective painkillers or anti-inflammatory drugs that do not usually cross-react with aspirin are codeine and low doses of acetaminophen or Tylenol. Some of the commonly used NSAID drugs that cross-react with aspirin are listed in Table 17.1.

TABLE 17.1
NSAID DRUGS THAT CROSS-REACT WITH ASPIRIN

GENERIC NAME	BRAND NAME
indomethacin	Indocin
fenoprofen	Nalfon
naproxen	Aleve, Naprosyn, Anaprox
tolmetin	Tolectin
ibuprofen	Motrin, Advil, Nuprin
mefenamic acid	Ponstel
sulindac	Clinoril
meclofenamate	Meclomen
piroxicam	Feldene
phenylbutazone	Butazolidin
flurbiprofen	Ansaid
ketoprofen	Orudis
diclofenac	Voltaren
diflunisal	Dolobid

Hundreds of non-prescription OTC (over-the-counter) medications contain aspirin or an NSAID drug, including Bufferin, Alka-Seltzer, Anacin, Pepto-Bismol, and many cough or cold preparations. Aspirin-sensitive asthmatics should compulsively read all drug labels in order to avoid hidden sources of aspirin or NSAIDs. Researchers from La Jolla, California, have shown that it is possible to desensitize people with aspirin or NSAID allergy. During this desensitization procedure, the aspirin-sensitive patient is given a tiny amount of aspirin that is progressively increased over a period of several hours or days. Once desensitized, the patient must take aspirin every day or the sensitivity to aspirin rapidly reappears.

In the late 1990s a new class of NSAIDs was marketed for victims of arthritic diseases. This class of drugs, known as the COX-2 inhibitors, blocks only one form of the enzyme cyclooxygenase, unlike aspirin which blocks both COX-1 and COX-2. While these new COX-2 drugs may not be that much more potent than aspirin, they have less of a tendency to cause gastritis and ulcers when taken on a long-term basis. Many reports have found that COX-2 drugs can be safely used in people with a history of aspirin or NSAID sensitivity. Our practice has carefully tested and successfully challenged several patients with a history of aspirin allergy or NSAID reactions with Vioxx, the new COX-2 inhibitor. The majority of our patients have tolerated these challenges without any adverse reactions. It should be emphasized that oral challenges with aspirin or any NSAID drug may induce severe bronchospasm and nasal reactions. Physicians conducting such challenges should be experienced in the proper techniques of challenge procedures and be prepared to aggressively treat allergic reactions or asthma attacks.

Doctors have always thought that NSAID-allergic people could safely take acetaminophen or Tylenol, but this may not be true. Dr. Guy Settipane has challenged fifty aspirin-sensitive asthmatics with 1,000- and 1,500-milligram doses of acetaminophen, and found that one-third reacted to the higher doses. Thus, it may be wise to avoid higher doses of Tylenol in aspirin-sensitive asthmatics.

Also, certain chemicals have been reported to cross-react with aspirin and the NSAID drugs. The most commonly cited chemical is Yellow Dye No. 5, or tartrazine, widely used to color foodstuffs, like butter, yellow. Many asthma specialists used to warn their aspirin-sensitive asthmatics to avoid yellow dye. Dr. Donald Stevenson put this myth to rest when none of 150 aspirin-sensitive asthmatics he challenged with tartrazine experienced any bronchospasm or nasal reactions. Thus aspirin-allergic or NSAID-sensitive asthmatics do not have to avoid tartrazine.

The Dangers of Occupational Asthma

In his *Affections,* Hippocrates wrote, "When you come to a patient's house you should ask what sort of pains he has, what causes them, how many days he has been sick, whether the bowels are working, and what sort of food he eats." In 1713, Bernadino Ramazzi, the father of occupational medicine, added one more important question to the medical history when he asked, "What occupation does he follow?" As early as the sixteenth century, researchers described asthmatic symptoms in grain handlers. Occupational asthma is defined as asthma due to causes and conditions attributable to a particular occupational environment and not to stimuli encountered outside the workplace. It is important to differentiate true occupational asthma from pre-existing asthma aggravated by an irritating or chemical exposure in the workplace.

There are two types of occupational asthma. The first and most common type occurs after prolonged exposure and allergic sensitization to the offending substance. The second form of occupational asthma occurs shortly after exposure to toxic levels of irritants, gases, and compounds not considered to be allergens. This form of occupational asthma is often called RAD, or "reactive airways disease."

It is estimated that more than two million Americans have occupational asthma. The exact number is difficult to pinpoint, as reporting guidelines vary from state to state. In many cases a wheezing worker is unwilling to report symptoms for fear of job loss. Job-related asthma is increasing in frequency and severity. More than three hundred different chemicals used in the workplace have been linked to asthma. Sometimes, asthma occurs immediately after starting work, whereas in other cases it may take months or years before the asthma symptoms surface. Both allergic and non-allergic substances trigger occupational asthma. In some cases, allergic asthma occurs when the worker is exposed to aeroallergens like plants, enzymes, or other biological agents.

The diagnosis of occupational asthma, while difficult to establish, is usually based on clinical history and appropriate lab and skin tests. Serial monitoring of lung functions in the workplace or direct bronchial challenges may be necessary to nail down the diagnosis. Occupational asthma has many disguises. A factory or office worker may report to work on Monday morning feeling well, only to suddenly develop a fever, chills, wheezing, or a flu-like illness that workers call the "Monday morning miseries." Other workers may have a delayed onset of symptoms, and they do not get sick until later in the week. Most people with occupational asthma improve on long holiday weekends or vacations. The triggers of occupational asthma include both the allergic and non-allergic materials. A typical non-allergic example of occupational asthma is the housewife who wheezes in her poorly ventilated laundry room when she inhales irritating ammonia or bleach fumes. An allergic example of occupational asthma would be the veterinary worker who wheezes when exposed to dogs or cats. Domestic cleaners are also prone to occupational asthma. A survey of house cleaners in Barcelona found that domestic cleaners were twice as likely to have asthma.

Compounds that induce occupational asthma can be broken down into two different groups based on their size or molecular weight. The high-molecular-weight group includes sensitizing proteins capable of eliciting a true allergic or IgE-mediated reaction. Such compounds include proteins like latex, enzymes, and plant products. One of the best examples of this form of occupational asthma is Baker's Asthma, where chefs and restaurant workers become allergic to wheat flour. In some forms of occupational asthma, workers are sensitized to minute amounts of chemicals used in the workplace. One of the most common examples of occupational asthma is TDI-induced asthma. TDI (toluene di-isocyanate) is a chemical widely used in the electronic and foam manufacturing industries. When released into the factory air in high concentrations, TDI is a potent irritant to the skin, nose, and lungs of normal individuals. Some workers have become sensitized to TDI when exposed to an air concentration as small as one part per billion.

The cause of TDI-induced asthma is poorly understood, as it is neither a simple irritant nor an allergic reaction. Heavy smokers and workers with a past history of asthma are more prone to TDI asthma. It may evolve into a very debilitating illness.

The treatment of occupational asthma is avoidance and environmental control. Employers must take appropriate steps to minimize or eliminate a worker's exposure to offending chemicals. One of the more successful models of industrial environmental control took place in the detergent industry. Dr. I. Leonard Bernstein from the University of Cincinnati discovered that detergent factory workers were developing asthma at an alarming rate. Bernstein's detective work revealed the asthma-inducer was an enzyme, *Bacilis subtilis,* which was added to the detergent to improve its stain-removing qualities. The detergent industry quickly responded to this threat and installed industrial environmental controls in their factories to minimize exposure to this enzyme. In 1970, it was estimated that one thousand of four thousand workers exposed to the detergent enzyme had developed sensitization to the chemical. By 1985, the number of cases had decreased to only one percent of exposed detergent workers. Detergent Worker's Asthma was virtually eliminated as an occupational health hazard.

Drug treatment of asthma is not an alternative to avoidance. However, when avoidance is impossible, pretreatment with asthma drugs may minimize the response to inhaled chemicals in the workplace. New data on occupational asthma implies that the damage to the lung may be permanent even when the worker is removed from the workplace. Thus, whenever possible, I now advise my patients with persistent asthma to get out of their work environment as soon as possible.

CHAPTER EIGHTEEN

Exercise-Induced Asthma (EIA)

EIA has intrigued physicians for more than two thousand years. In A.D. 200, Aretaeus stated, "If from running or gymnastic exercise or any other work, the breathing becomes difficult, it is called asthma." In 1864, H. A. Salter, who recognized that cold air triggered asthma, speculated that the passage of fresh and cold air over the bronchial mucosa triggered asthma by irritating the nervous system.

These accurate descriptions of EIA have stood the test of time. Jim Davis, the creator of the cartoon cat Garfield, attributes his artistic talent to having to spend most of his childhood drawing indoors because of his asthma. Other creative artists whose success may have been helped by their asthma include Ludwig van Beethoven, Charles Dickens, and Robert Louis Stevenson.

Sports-Induced Asthma (EIA)

Many surveys in young athletes with questionnaires, physical exams, and exercise challenges found that EIA is a widely under-diagnosed condition. Dr. Margaret Guill found that 13 percent of surveyed athletes in Georgia had EIA, a much higher rate than previously reported in college and Olympic athletes.

Most, if not all, people with asthma cough or wheeze when they exercise, especially when they exercise in cold, dry air. This syndrome has various names, including EIA, exercise-induced bronchospasm, and sports-induced asthma. The duration and intensity of any exercise activity is governed by one's physical conditioning and endurance level. During exercise, the bronchial tubes normally open up or dilate to improve the exchange of oxygen and carbon dioxide. This dilation of the bronchial tubes is due to release of adrenaline from the adrenal gland. Just the opposite occurs when an asthmatic exercises. The bronchial tubes tighten and, within five to ten minutes after starting exercise, the exercising asthmatic starts to cough or wheeze.

While some individuals are able to continue exercising or "run through their attack," others must stop exercising altogether. Sometimes the asthma symptoms do not begin until after exercise is completed. A few people do not cough or wheeze until several hours after exercising. This is called delayed EIA. Most attacks of EIA subside within thirty to sixty minutes, even when untreated. Several factors, including climate and the type of exercise, influence the severity of EIA. Exercising in cold, dry air is much more likely to trigger asthma than exercising in warm, humid air. Running is more asthmagenic than swimming or cycling. The duration of exercise is also important. A longer exercise period increases the likelihood of EIA. Many people with EIA only wheeze during the allergy season or during periods of high temperatures and humidity when air pollution levels are high.

EIA is essentially a mini-asthma attack, and for some people it may be their only form of asthma. Whenever I confront a patient with asthma who does not cough or wheeze with exercise, I will closely question the diagnosis of asthma. When exercise is the only asthma trigger, I often use the medical term exercise-induced bronchospasm, not EIA. Putting the buzzword "asthma" into a medical report or insurance form may result in that person being declared ineligible for entrance into the armed forces, flight schools, or service academies, or raise the premiums of health or life insurance coverage.

Mechanisms of Exercise-Induced Asthma

Inhaled air is normally humidified and warmed to body temperature by the time it reaches the lung. By testing people with asthma in laboratory settings, researchers have learned that when asthmatics hyperventilate during exercise, they do not warm or humidify their inspired air as well as non-asthmatics. Thus, they inhale dry, colder air that acts as a potent bronchoconstricter. This explains why EIA is more likely to occur while jogging outdoors on a cold winter morning, versus swimming indoors in a well-humidified pool. The exact location of this temperature and humidity defect is unknown.

The swelling of the nasal passages and increased secretions in exercise, especially in cold air, also limit airflow and warming of the lower airways. These important observations have led to very simple advice for athletes who have asthma, especially wintertime joggers. Wear a protective mask or scarf over your mouth and nose when exercising in cold dry weather! This allows you to rebreathe warmer, more humid, expired air.

Diagnosis of EIA

The diagnosis of EIA is usually quite easy. The basic question I ask my patients is, "Do you cough or wheeze when you exert yourself, especially in colder, dry weather?" When the answer is yes, the diagnosis of EIA is almost a certainty. Sometimes physiologic shortness of breath or simply being out of shape may be confused with EIA, and an exercise challenge may be necessary.

I sometimes conduct an informal exercise challenge where a patient is seen in the office, and a baseline lung function and a chest exam are performed. The patient then runs outdoors (weather permitting) for a period of five to ten minutes and returns to the office for a reexamination and breathing test. The presence of wheezing or a drop of

15 to 20 percent or more in one-second vital capacity (FEV1) or peak expiratory flow rate usually confirms the diagnosis of EIA. Such a free-run challenge may be more asthmagenic than a laboratory treadmill test, as it can be conducted in the real-life outdoor setting of cool, dry air. The diagnosis of EIA can be made at home or on the athletic field by measuring their peak flow rates before and after exercise. Exercise challenges in adults with known or suspected cardiovascular disease should only be performed in laboratory facilities with the capability of monitoring heart rate and blood pressure.

One condition that may be confused with EIA is exercise-induced laryngeal stridor. This condition is more common among top trained, young female athletes who develop stridor or a croupy-like breathing pattern during maximal exercise. Unlike those athletes with true EIA, they do not cough or wheeze during or after exercise.

Taking a Closer Look: Sports-Induced Asthma

Is EIA being over-diagnosed in the general population, especially in children and adolescents? In my opinion the answer is definitely yes. Most individuals, except highly conditioned athletes, become short of breath during vigorous aerobic exercise. The degree of shortness of breath is directly related to one's endurance or physical conditioning. Over the past decade, I have seen a growing number of people, usually children or young adults, referred for evaluation of exercise or "sports-induced asthma." These children and young adults often have no other signs of asthma, such as coughing or wheezing when exposed to allergens or during respiratory infections.

The typical patient with sports-induced asthma is usually an active junior high or high school athlete—more often a soccer player. These people are frequently accompanied to the office by their father who, as luck may have it, is also the kid's coach. Dad relates that his child, who has been active in a sport such as soccer for several years, can no longer run as fast or as long as his or her teammates. After competing in vigorous activities for eight to ten minutes, this youngster develops a shortness of breath that limits performance level. The under-performing athlete has usually seen their primary-care provider, who without the benefit of an exercise challenge or a lung function test, makes a snap diagnosis of "sports-induced asthma" and prescribes an asthma inhaler. When these student-athletes did not respond to the inhaler and athletic performance does not improve, they are often referred for further evaluation.

Most people with "sports-induced asthma" rarely cough or wheeze, and they have no other allergy problems like hay fever or eczema. The proper approach to these people is to take a careful history, perform a breathing test before and after inhaling a bronchodilator, and do an exercise challenge. Sometimes it may be necessary to perform a methacholine challenge test. Between visits, the patient is told to record the peak flow reading before, during, and after exercise. The diagnosis of sports-induced asthma should be discarded when the evaluation fails to show any evidence of EIA.

Most children experience a growth spurt in late childhood and adolescence. This growth spurt is accompanied by a substantial increase in height and weight. This means that it takes more endurance and physical conditioning to perform at a higher level of competition. Soccer is a particularly strenuous sport, as it involves free running outdoors, often in cold, dry air. It also is a sport with no time-outs or rest periods. Over the past decade, soccer has grown in popularity. In many cities and towns hundreds of young children start playing soccer at an early age. As children grow older and enter high school, the level of competition intensifies and team selection becomes more competitive. Only the very best and fastest players are chosen for the "select teams." This pyramid effect leads to significant fallout, and disappointed parents begin looking for medical reasons why their child can no longer run as fast and as long as the better players. In my opinion this is a major reason for the over-diagnosis of sports-induced asthma.

Treatment of EIA

EIA can usually be effectively treated. Warming up before exercise will reduce the intensity of EIA. This is based on the observation that exercise challenges performed sixty minutes after exercise produce less bronchoconstriction than the first exercise period. A warm-down exercise may also decrease the degree of delayed EIA. Individuals with EIA who are engaged in intensive competition should perform light exercises every thirty to forty minutes when there are long intervals between events. Avoiding a quick return to a cold environment after exercising in warm air (or vice versa) also lowers the degree of EIA. In my college days in New Hampshire, I always wheezed after I left the gymnasium and went out into the cold New Hampshire winter air.

You should should try to exercise indoors when air pollutant levels are high. Wear a mask or scarf when exercising in colder air. Nasal breathing is not recommended during intense exercise, as most athletes do not move enough air through their nose to meet the high oxygen requirements of aerobic exercise. Dr. Robert Strunk evaluated the fitness of children with asthma at the National Jewish Hospital in Denver and found that most asthmatic children at this institution were very much out of shape. Strunk found that people with asthma could improve their performance in activities such as bicycling, running, and swimming by improving their physical fitness.

The most effective medicine in relieving and preventing EIA is the beta-agonist drug albuterol (Proventyl) or pirbuterol (Maxair), which prevents or reduces bronchospasm for up to two hours when taken ten to fifteen minutes before exercise. When albuterol or pirbuterol does not work, I add cromolyn sodium (Intal) thirty to sixty minutes before exercise to block or minimize EIA. Inhaled cortisone drugs do not reduce EIA if administered as a single dose before exercise, but they may minimize EIA when administered over an extended period.

People who do not respond to albuterol, pirbuterol, or Intal can try either Serevent or Singulair. While this two-pronged approach may help asthmatics who vigorously exercise more than once a day or for longer periods of time, due to the potential risks of using a long-acting, beta-agonist drug as monotherapy, I only recommend this combination in people who are taking inhaled cortisone on a daily basis. Thus, when all these therapies fail to control EIA, it may be necessary to use an inhaled cortisone drug.

Rich Dumont and Marax

Years ago, Olympians who took asthma drugs during competition were severely penalized. In 1972, USA swimmer Rich Dumont forfeited his 400-meter gold medal when it was discovered that he had taken an older asthma medication (Marax) before his race. Unfortunately, Marax contained ephedrine, a known nervous system stimulant that is banned from Olympic competition. Dumont's misfortune forced the Olympic Committee to change its rules. Dumont should be awarded a much larger medal by society for alerting the world to the plight of the asthmatic athlete and showing just what an athlete who had asthma could accomplish.

Asthma medication use in the 1998 Winter Olympics ranged from a high of 60 percent in cross-country skiers to a low of 3 percent for bobsledders. The International Olympic Committee (IOC) now feels that it is quite possible that some athletes are using asthma medicines as performance-enhancing drugs, especially the beta-agonist drugs, which are classified as stimulants. In August 2000, the IOC toughened up its requirements for the use of asthma medications. Athletes must now provide clinical and laboratory evidence that they have asthma, including lung function tests, before competing. These tests will be reviewed and approved by a panel of medical experts.

The Medical Commission of the IOC has approved and banned certain drugs which are listed in Table 18.1.

TABLE 18.1
IOC ASTHMA AND ALLERGY MEDICATIONS

ALLOWED TO USE
- Sodium cromolyn (Intal) or nedocromil (Tilade)
- Leukotriene modifiers
- Ipratropium bromide (Atrovent)
- Theophylline
- Antihistamines

PERMITTED BY NOTIFICATION
- Inhaled albuterol (Proventil, Ventolin), salmeterol (Severent)
- Inhaled cortisone drugs

STRICTLY PROHIBITED
- Systemic or oral corticosteroids
- Other inhaled beta-agonists than those noted above
- Systemic or oral beta-agonists
- Inhaled or systemic EpiPen

Readers who wish to learn more about EIA should read *Asthma and Exercise* (Henry Holt and Co., 1990). Written by Nancy Hogshead and Gerald Cousens, this fine book details the asthma experiences of Nancy Hogshead, an asthmatic who won four Olympic medals in swimming at the 1984 Summer Olympics. Hogshead vividly explains that she had undiagnosed asthma up until the 1984 Olympics. It was not uncommon for her to develop shortness of breath and coughing after a race. She simply thought she had small lungs. After finishing fourth in the 200-meter butterfly, Hogshead was short of breath and began to cough. A nearby doctor asked her if she always coughed like that after a race and suggested that she possibly had asthma. After she returned to Duke University, lung function tests determined that she did have EIA. Hogshead's book convincingly demonstrates how essential it is for a patient or family to take control of EIA and not be controlled by it. The authors present clear and detailed advice on how adults and children with asthma can cope with exercise and sports. Hogshead and Cousens describe the asthma experiences of several famous athletes who took control of their asthma and went on to high achievement, including Jackie Joyner-Kersee, Mike Gminski, Danny Manning, Jim Ryan, Cheryl Durstin-Decker, and Sam Perkins.

Scuba Diving and Asthma

The term scuba, which is the abbreviation for self-contained underwater breathing apparatus, describes the diving apparatus that allows divers to carry their own air supply. Scuba diving became a worldwide recreational activity after modern scuba gear was developed by Jacques Cousteau and Emile Gagnon in 1943. Now there are over six million certified divers in the United States.

The most common reason for a death during scuba diving is drowning. The second most common cause of death is arterial gas embolism. When divers ascend to the surface, the volume of air in their lung expands. If the diver ascends too quickly, air cannot be exhaled fast enough and it is forced into the arteries supplying blood to the lung. When air bubbles enter the blood stream, they cause an air embolism to other organs of the body, including the brain. Air may also leak into tissues surrounding the lung and cause a pneumothorax or collapse of the lung. This condition occurs because increased pressure causes more nitrogen to be dissolved in the blood. When the diver comes up too quickly, the increased nitrogen reverts to its gaseous state, causing nitrogen bubbles. The end result is called decompression sickness or "the bends." In milder cases, symptoms consist of localized joint pain and skin rashes, whereas in more serious cases air embolism to the brain and spinal cord can lead to paralysis and death.

What is the risk of diving if you have asthma? It is commonly agreed that symptomatic asthma is a contraindication to diving due to exercise limitations and mucus plugging. Air trapped in the lungs may predispose the asthmatic to an air embolism on ascent to the surface. The bottom line is that asthmatics who are coughing or wheezing should not dive.

What about asthmatics who are not having symptoms? Several surveys by popular diving magazines uncovered hundreds of divers with asthma who reported that they dove on a regular basis with little or no problems. Older recommendations cautioned that asthmatics with a history of active asthma within the past five years should not dive. More recent publications reported that people with normal lung functions and little airway reactivity in response to exercise or cold air have no greater risk for barotrauma than normal subjects. The recommendations regarding the risks of scuba diving in asthmatics are sketchy and conflicting. ACAAI (American College of Allergy, Asthma and Immunology) guidelines for scuba diving state the following:

- Any individual with active asthma should refrain from diving even if their lung functions are normal.
- Persons with a remote history of asthma who are completely without asthma symptoms and have normal lung functions can probably safely engage in diving.
- Persons with a vague history of asthma should be examined and studied before being allowed to dive.

Dr. Arthur Torre, an asthma specialist and avid diver, is a member of PADI or the Professional Association of Diving Instructors. PADI and other diving organizations had formerly stated that asthma was an absolute contraindication to diving. In 1995, Dr. Torre and his fellow diving physicians reviewed the data on this issue and came up with the new recommendation that asthma was a relative contraindication to diving: if your asthma was not well controlled, you should not dive. Under current guidelines, most diving organizations, including the Underseas Hyperbaric Medical Society, state that to dive safely, an asthmatic should have normal lung functions before and after exercise.

The data collected by the Divers Alert Network found that divers with asthma have no greater risk for air embolism than nonasthmatics. Dr. Torre recommends measuring lung functions before and after exercise and monitoring lung functions with a peak flow meter twice a day for a few weeks before diving and during a diving trip. When lung functions are normal and the patient has no asthma symptoms, Dr. Torre feels the chances of having asthma problems while diving are relatively small.

I agree with Dr. Torre. If you have active, persistent, uncontrolled asthma, you should not dive. Individuals with controlled asthma should be evaluated by lung function tests and seek authorization from qualified physicians before diving. If you have mild intermittent asthma with normal lung function tests, diving is probably safe. Pre-dive administration of a short-acting bronchodilator will minimize the risk of bronchospasm during a dive. Asthmatics who dive should also be checked and treated for ear and nasal-sinus problems, as barotrauma of the middle ear and sinus cavities is the most common medical complication in divers.

For further information on diving and asthma, contact the Divers Alert Network at Duke University in North Carolina (1-800-445-2671 or www.diversalertnetwork.org).

CHAPTER NINETEEN

Childhood and Young Adult Asthma

Asthma is a common childhood illness. Studies from England, Australia, Canada, and the United States suggest that one child in ten has asthma. Pediatric asthma is the most frequent reason for missed school days and emergency room visits in pediatric centers. Asthma accounts for one in every four pediatric asthma admissions to inner-city hospitals, and produces more in-hospital days than any other childhood disease.

One-third of children who develop asthma do so before their third birthday, and nearly 80 percent of all asthmatic children start to wheeze before they enter the first grade. The sex distribution changes with age. Asthmatic boys outnumber girls in early childhood. In middle childhood, the sex ratio evens out, whereas in adolescence females outnumber males by a three to two margin.

The Wheezing Infant

Asthma specialists now know that asthma is a common disease of infancy and early childhood. Doctors at the Mayo Clinic studied the medical records of the residents of Homestead County, Minnesota. They found that 60 percent of all asthmatics of any age had been diagnosed by age three, and almost 90 percent had developed asthma by age six. It is easy to both over-diagnose and under-diagnose asthma in infancy and early childhood. The first one or two episodes of a wheezing illness in infancy are usually called wheezy bronchitis or bronchiolitis by the family doctor or pediatrician. Nearly 50 percent of infants experience a transient wheezing illness from time to time because of the small size of their airways. When children grow, their airways enlarge and many outgrow the tendency to wheeze when they have a respiratory infection. Doctors have to be careful not to over-treat infants who have two or three bouts of transient wheezing, as many do not develop full-blown asthma. Only one-third of wheezy infants go on to develop persistent wheezing or true asthma. One of the more blatant examples of over-treatment occurs when an infant or toddler has his or her first episode of wheezing. Many family physicians and pediatricians jump the gun and prescribe a nebulizer for home administration of bronchodilators. Not only is this overkill from a treatment standpoint, it is economically unsound, as many of these children never experience another bout of wheezing, and unused and expensive nebulizers simply gather dust in the closet.

Sometimes the diagnostic pendulum swings the other way. When an infant or young child experiences three or more episodes of a wheezing-type illness, the likelihood of asthma increases. The correct diagnosis of asthma is often delayed, as many doctors are unwilling to put the word "asthma" into play. Doctors call it persistent wheezing, bronchitis, or bronchiolitis, as using the word "asthma" implies that the child may have a chronic disease that might last several years or even a lifetime.

The hesitancy of doctors to label a wheezing youngster as having asthma is not unique to America. Doctor L. Hey of Tyneside, England, found that 11 percent of all the children in his town had asthma symptoms, yet only one in three was prescribed appropriate asthma medicines and only one in ten parents knew their child had asthma. The salient point here is that reluctance by doctors to use the term asthma can lead to delayed, inappropriate, and poor care.

I fully concur with Hey's observations. I have evaluated scores of children who have been coughing and wheezing for many years, yet the diagnosis of asthma has never been entertained. Parents are totally shocked when the diagnosis of asthma is brought up. Doctors have told the parents that their child is "bronchial," a misnomer that leads to under-treatment of a very treatable condition. In summary, any infant or child who experiences three or more episodes of wheezy bronchitis may have asthma. The diagnosis of asthma is almost a certainty when a child persistently coughs or wheezes between respiratory infections, during exercise, or while sleeping.

How Childhood Asthma Develops

The potential for developing asthma and other allergic diseases at a young age depends upon one's genetic make-up combined with environmental exposures that send the immune system down the allergy-prone Th2 pathway. What is the natural history for the unfortunate infant born with the asthma-allergy genetic coding? Susceptible infants will first develop a scaly, itchy skin rash called eczema or atopic dermatitis. Next, they experience an allergic reaction to milk or eggs. Typical symptoms of food allergy in infancy include colic, vomiting, diarrhea, or hives. The child who hits for the cycle will eventually develop allergic rhinitis (hay fever) and asthma.

An infant has a higher risk of developing asthma if a food allergy or eczema appears before three months of age. The first hint of the disease is wheezing or chest congestion during a respiratory infection. Most milk and egg food allergies are outgrown by age four or five, only to be replaced by the development of allergies to inhaled allergens such as dust mites, molds, household pets, and pollens. The exception to this food allergy scenario is the young child with peanut or tree nut allergy, which can persist for years or a lifetime.

Do environmental controls and dietary precautions by the mother during pregnancy or while breastfeeding prevent the development of asthma in their offspring? Several investigators have attempted to answer this difficult question. Doctor Robert Zeiger of San Diego divided high-risk families and their mothers into a prevention and a control group. The mothers in the prevention group avoided allergenic foods during pregnancy and while breastfeeding. They were asked to eliminate pets and institute strict dust-mite controls within their home. The control group made no changes in their diet or lifestyle. While the incidence of food allergy and eczema was much lower in the prevention group in infancy and early childhood, the rate of allergy and asthma was the same in both groups by age four. While maternal environmental precautions and avoidance of allergenic foods lowered the incidence of food allergy and eczema in early childhood, these measures did not prevent children from eventually developing allergies or asthma later on in childhood.

It is fairly easy to identify those infants who may develop true asthma later on in childhood. The high-risk children have food (egg or milk) allergy or eczema at an early age (before age three), a family history of asthma or allergy, mothers who smoke, and high levels of IgE antibody or eosinophils. Is allergy skin testing of any value in early infancy in these children? One myth perpetuated by pediatricians and family physicians is that infants and young children with eczema or food allergy are too young to undergo skin tests, as skin tests are not very reliable in this age group. Nothing could be further from the truth.

Skin testing is an easy and reliable way to pick out those youngsters at risk to develop additional allergies or asthma. Why do allergy skin tests in an infant or a young child who has had an obvious reaction to milk or eggs? When the clinical history is consistent with a food reaction, I may not test for that specific food. The main reason to do limited skin tests to other foods and allergens in this age group is that you may uncover unidentified allergies and implement preventive dietary and environmental precautions. The other reason for skin tests in this age group is to rule out allergy and minimize unnecessary and sometimes expensive environmental precautions. I frequently encounter young children with negative skin tests whose parents have already removed family pets and have spent hundreds of dollars on unnecessary environmental precautions within the home.

Late-Onset Childhood Asthma

Sometimes asthma may not begin until later on in childhood. A Melbourne, Australia, asthma study found that almost all early transient wheezers were wheeze-free by twelve years of age. Most children with only a few episodes of wheezing had a benign course whereas children with persistent asthma at age ten had significant wheezing in adulthood. Wheezing episodes during viral infections that began after age three were rarely troublesome. Nearly 50 percent of Australian children in this study stopped wheezing by the age of ten, and very few had persistent asthma in adulthood.

Risk Factors for Persistent Adult Asthma
- Family history of asthma-allergy (especially in the mother)
- Male sex
- Exposure to RSV virus
- Tobacco smoke exposure
- Atopic dermatitis
- Food allergy to egg or milk in the first year of life
- Lower socioeconomic status
- Early exposure to mites, molds, or cockroaches
- Obesity
- Wheezing at age ten or eleven years of age

It is now clear that persistent asthma is associated with a well-defined set of risk factors. Older children (aged eight to eleven years) with persistent wheezing have more severe symptoms, lower lung functions, and more allergy problems. In the Australian study, early-onset asthma often predicted chronic asthma that persisted into adult life. In these people, the most troublesome period was between the ages of eight and fourteen, when asthma symptoms persisted for months at a time. Many of these children were seldom wheeze-free. The majority were males who were highly reactive to airway challenges. Only five percent of these children were wheeze-free as adults, although boys seemed to improve more during puberty than girls. Lung function levels were significantly lower in this group when compared with those with infrequent episodic asthma.

More importantly, there is mounting evidence that most of the deterioration in lung function seen in older children and adults with asthma occurs in early school years. Most children who develop persistent wheezing start life with normal lung functions. By the age of six, the persistent wheezers have significant deterioration in lung function as compared with children who are wheeze-free. It appears that the persistent bronchial reactivity characteristic of chronic asthma may alter lung development during the period of fastest lung growth—between birth and age seven. Whether the poor lung function observed in these children is associated with severe asthma or is only a marker of severe asthma is unknown. It is imperative that children who fall into this high-risk group be promptly diagnosed and aggressively treated at an early age. Proper asthma treatment in the high-risk preschool child may prevent permanent remodeling or lung scarring and a lifetime of asthma.

Adolescent-Onset Asthma

When asthma begins in adolescence, the outlook is not so rosy. This type of asthma is more common in girls and is likely to be a non-allergic form of asthma with less chance of a remission, especially in females. A survey in the Mississippi River Valley looking at junior high and high school students found that 16 percent had asthma. Girls had more asthma than boys, and their asthma was more severe than that found in the male students. Young adults with asthma pose a special challenge to asthma care providers. Adolescent-onset asthma is often quite severe and can be difficult to control. The teenage years can be a bumpy road on the path to adulthood. Peer pressure can lead to non-compliance and disease denial on the part of young adults with asthma. A large number of adolescents with undiagnosed asthma fail to get care. A survey of 122,829 children in North Carolina schools found that 6 percent had undiagnosed asthma. Adolescent-onset asthma is likely to persist into adulthood and cause a permanent loss of lung function, especially in adolescent smokers. Near-fatal and fatal asthma attacks are more common in young adults than children. Kids might overuse rescue inhalers, fail to take anti-inflammatory medicine on a regular basis, smoke, and disregard the effect of the environment. Special educational efforts are needed to ensure compliance with medication programs and identification and avoidance of asthma triggers. Adolescents should be encouraged to take charge of their asthma action plans.

Will My Child Outgrow Asthma?

One of the more commonly asked questions by parents of asthmatic children is, "Will my child outgrow asthma?" I used to tell parents that it was a coin toss—one-third outgrew their disease, one-third got better, and one-third did not improve. New epidemiological studies offer a more promising outlook for childhood asthma. The majority of children below three years of age who only wheeze with respiratory infections stop wheezing by mid-childhood. Among 2,345 children in the United Kingdom who wheezed before five years of age, 80 percent were wheeze-free by age ten. The more wheezing episodes before age five, the less chance the child had of outgrowing asthma. Ninety-two percent of children with one wheezing episode before age five were symptom-free at age ten.

Long-term follow-up studies suggest that most children with asthma improve during adolescence, and up to 50 percent are wheeze-free in adulthood. Nevertheless, about 80 percent of symptom-free young adults still have evidence of a twitchy lung or bronchial reactivity and may redevelop asthma at any time in adulthood. Thus, having childhood asthma significantly increases one's risk of redeveloping asthma as an adult, especially if the first attack occurred after age two or if there were more than ten attacks during childhood.

Recurrent Croup and General Anesthesia

Two additional conditions that may be risk factors for childhood asthma are repeated bouts of croup and exposure to general anesthesia. Many children experience recurrent croup throughout childhood. Some of these children are seven to eight years of age, well beyond the classic age for croup. I have had some personal experience with this problem, as my oldest daughter, whose twin brother has asthma, had numerous episodes of croup up until age twelve. I never really associated croup with asthma, but it appears that some croupy children have a form of asthma that only affects their large airways. A study in Belgium found that a high percentage of children with asthma had recurrent croup. The Belgian investigators found a strong association between a positive family history of asthma and croup. If recurrent croup is indeed a unique form of asthma, the good news is that most children will outgrow it as my daughter did. Dr. Douglas Johnestone of Rochester, N.Y., reported that children subjected to general anesthesia at a young age had a much greater chance of developing asthma. This paper was of particular interest to me. My oldest son, who developed asthma at age four, underwent a rather difficult hernia repair at age two that required nearly two hours of general anesthesia.

The Critical Role of Parents and Caretakers

At-risk families must learn as much as possible about controlling asthma. This includes being able to identify warning symptoms, understanding asthma triggers and asthma medications, and having a sound asthma action plan to put into place when asthma relapses occur. Everyone involved in the care of the child must understand these plans.

Babysitters

The following set of guidelines was developed by the American Lung Association to help responsible parents be comfortable leaving the care of an asthmatic child to caretakers or babysitters:

- Use babysitters who will follow directions and comply with a simple asthma action plan.
- The babysitter does not have to be an expert in asthma care.
- Do not employ babysitters who smoke.
- Provide proper training and education, including a list of asthma medications and asthma triggers to avoid.
- Babysitters must know how to administer medications, especially when younger children require nebulizers.
- Encourage the babysitter to treat your child no differently than other children.
- Provide a written asthma action plan that includes where parents can be contacted and emergency phone numbers of your doctor and local hospital.

School

Asthma is the leading cause for school absenteeism. Nearly six million schoolchildren have asthma, and lost school days number over five hundred thousand each year. Make sure the school your child attends meets the following conditions:

- Provides an equal opportunity for a normal learning experience.
- Does not allow students to feel sickly or different.

- Allows participation in all physical activities up to the student's physical capacity.
- Guarantees medical support during acute attacks of asthma.

The School Nurse

The school nurse is the team captain who plays the leading role in developing a health-care plan for students with asthma. The school nurse should:

- Meet with parents to assess asthma triggers in the home environment.
- Review the student's asthma treatment program and action plan.
- Monitor early warning signs of unstable asthma and use peak flow meters.
- Assume responsibility for educating teachers and physical education instructors about allergy and asthma.
- Take responsibility to minimize the exposure to allergens or irritants in the students' classrooms and ensure they follow specially prescribed diets in the school cafeteria. Students with peanut or tree nut allergy require extra supervision, as most near-fatal or fatal allergic reactions to peanuts and nuts occur outside the home.
- Allow students to use asthma medicines, and permit students to self-medicate when fully authorized by parents and the physician.
- Stay in close contact with physical education instructors to ensure fair grading for students with allergies and exercise-induced asthma.

The Classroom Teacher

The classroom teacher is in the best position to observe the student's daily progress from a health and educational standpoint. The class-room teacher should:

- Be provided with information and educated about asthma and the side effects of asthma medications.
- Inform the school nurse and parents if the student has a significant deterioration in school performance or develops behavioral problems.
- Keep the classroom relatively dust-free and not allow furry or feathered animals in the students' environment.
- Be prepared to handle an acute asthma attack.
- Allow the student extra time to make up missed work or exams due to absences.
- Treat the student as a normal human being and provide a normal learning experience.
- Minimize chalk dust exposure by using a wet cloth or sponge, not an eraser, to clean blackboards.
- Be aware that asthma is a very treatable condition.

One role of the classroom teacher may involve environmental control. Emerging evidence implies that exposure to animals, especially cat allergen, in the classroom can trigger asthma in students who do not have cats in their home. Simply seating the cat-allergic child away from students who have cats at home may prevent cat-induced wheezing in the school classroom. In day care or nursery settings where children spend a lot of time playing on the floor or in traditional classroom settings, removing or limiting allergen-laden carpeting may be helpful.

The Role of the Coach and Physical Education Instructors

Physical education instructors and coaches have a unique opportunity to impact the life of a student with asthma by encouraging active participation in gym and sports activities. Physical education instructors and coaches should:

- Be provided with education detailing the telltale signs and symptoms of asthma and allergic conditions.
- Permit and encourage the student to participate in regular physical activities.
- Notify parents if the student cannot fully participate in gym. Do not allow the student to stop taking gym classes unless so directed by a doctor.
- Allow for a reduction in outdoor activities during cold weather or periods of air pollution. Excuse the student from classes if he or she has significant asthma symptoms.
- Attempt to determine the child's physical limitations. Encourage the child to function within those limits.
- Not attempt to force the student to exceed his or her limitations, such as running laps outdoors on a cold day, when such activity is likely to trigger asthma. Encourage warm-up activities and exercises.
- Become familiar with exercises that are best tolerated by the student with asthma.
- Allow the student to set his or her pace on a daily basis.
- Permit the student to take the prescribed asthma drugs before or during exercise, including after-school activities like games or practices, with no inconvenience.

The Asthma and Allergy Foundation of America (AAFA) has developed an Asthma Action Card for asthma. These AAFA cards allow the physician and the family to provide clear, concise information on triggers, prevention, and emergency treatment. This card outlines the patient's basic allergies and common asthma triggers, and lists a medication plan that utilizes peak flow readings. In the opinion of many school nurses in the National Association of School Nurses, the size of the asthma and allergy population in schools is increasing.

The Use of Inhalers in School

One of the major problems encountered by a student with asthma is that many schools do not allow them to carry their own asthma medicines or inhalers and assume responsibility for their own care. The most frequent indication for an asthma medicine in the school setting will be exercise-induced asthma. When a school prohibits the student with asthma from self-medicating with an asthma inhaler, the student must then go to the school office or nursing station before or after a gym class or exercise period to get the inhaler to prevent or relieve exercise-induced asthma. This is both an embarrassment and a great inconvenience for the student. In large schools, the gym class may be completed by the time the student returns from the nursing office. Under such circumstances, most asthmatic students will only go to the school office or the nursing station in an emergency situation. Not only is this unfair, it is a violation of one's rights, as the student is being deprived of his or her basic rights to fully participate in everyday school activities.

The Drug Committee of the American Academy of Allergy, Asthma and Immunology studied this problem and published a position statement that encourages schools to allow responsible students of any age to keep inhalers in their possession and assume responsibility for self-management with asthma inhalers.

Preparing the Student for the School Year

A report by the Allergy and Asthma Network—Mothers of Asthmatics nicely outlines the appropriate steps to take to approach asthma in the school setting. Proper communication and information sharing is the best way to minimize parental concerns. Parents should meet with the school nurse, teachers, or administrators before the school year begins.

If the child has food allergies, the cafeteria manager should be included. The important topics to discuss in such a meeting include:

- The student's allergy and asthma medical history.
- The goal of any treatment plan.
- How to identify and handle emergencies.
- How to use allergy and asthma medications.
- How to use spacers, peak flow meters, and EpiPen.
- Who to contact during the school day.
- The student's ability to self-medicate.
- A list of food allergies and asthma triggers.
- A plan to make up missed school work.

Any problems you may experience are usually solved when you remind administrators, teachers, or gym instructors that students with asthma are protected by federal law under section 504 of the Rehabilitation Act of 1973, the Individuals with Disabilities Education Act.

Parents whose children do not receive proper support from school authorities should inform them that they plan to file a formal complaint with the state department of education or the regional office of the United States Department of Education—Office for Civil Rights. In my experience this approach solves most, if not all, discriminatory problems in the school setting.

When the Student Leaves Home

When the asthmatic student leaves home for the first time to attend school or college or to travel, special steps need to be taken to build a solid foundation for asthma self-management. The departing student, who will be independent for the first time in his or her life, should have a sound grasp of the fundamentals of asthma therapy. He or she should know how to use medications and when to seek additional care for acute asthma.

The student's physician or asthma doctor should prepare a summary of the student's medical history and a current list of medications that allows school health-care providers unfamiliar with the student's medical background to follow an asthma treatment program. The student's doctor should also write a letter to school housing authorities requesting non-allergenic bedding, non-smoking roommates, and air-conditioned dormitories. Many boarding schools and colleges are situated in remote, rural areas where competent asthma care may not be readily available. The student should be encouraged to communicate by phone with parents or doctors during an asthma flare-up.

As many students tend to neglect their medications and environmental controls during their first semester, I usually schedule a brief follow-up visit during a vacation period to make sure they are following their treatment program. Many parents, including me, have noted that school dorms or apartments are potential dust bins. Fortunately, they often have less carpeting and upholstered furniture and no exposure to dogs or cats. Therefore, many dust-mite and pet-allergic students experience dramatic improvement during their first few months away from home. Some students are able to stop daily asthma medications once they move from their dust-mite- and pet-allergen-infested homes. A severe relapse is not uncommon when they return home for the Thanksgiving or Christmas holidays. Re-exposure to a homestead with high levels of dust mites or dog or cat allergen is usually the cause of such holiday asthma relapses.

Key Steps for Savvy College Students
- Whenever possible, choose an air-conditioned dormitory.
- Keep room furniture to a minimum.
- Bring your own pillow.
- Avoid dusty upholstered furniture and old rugs.
- Use dust-mite-proof covers on your pillow and mattress.
- Hot wash your bedding weekly.

- Use HEPA air purifiers.
- Prohibit smoking in your room.
- Keep pets out of your room.
- Keep a list of your asthma medications.
- Do not stop taking your asthma medications.
- Have an asthma action plan.
- Develop a medication kit for "road trips."
- Avoid "all nighters" before exams.
- Continue allergy shots at the school health facility.
- Get an annual flu shot.
- If needed, know when and where to find an asthma specialist.

CHAPTER TWENTY

Asthma in Women

There is a gathering body of evidence that age and sex strongly influence the risk for developing asthma. In early puberty, the sex ratio of asthma gradually evens out. In young adulthood, the pendulum dramatically shifts with asthma becoming more common and more severe in women—a pattern that persists throughout adulthood. In a Tucson, Arizona, study, the incidence of adult-onset asthma was twice as common in females versus males. This sexual trend is most pronounced in women over forty. There is a wide gender disparity in the severity of asthma at various ages. Young boys (under age ten) are twice as likely as girls of that age to require hospitalizations, whereas adult women are three times more likely than men to be hospitalized. Adult women are hospitalized for longer periods of time, and are more prone to near-fatal and fatal asthma episodes. The reasons for this striking difference in the incidence and severity of asthma in adolescent and adult women are poorly understood. The possibilities include genetic factors, hormonal imbalances, and increased exposure to indoor allergens.

Premenstrual Asthma

Hormonal factors undoubtedly play a key role in asthma. Up to 40 percent of asthmatic women experience an increase in their asthma symptoms prior to and during their menstrual period. One emergency room survey found that four times as many women sought emergency room care before or during their menstrual cycle. The authors of this paper speculated that a rapid decline in circulating estrogen prior to menses predisposed women to an asthma relapse. Conflicting reports have found that hormonal replacement both improves and worsens asthma. Thus, at this time it is impossible to make any recommendations on the use or nonuse of hormone replacement therapy in post-menopausal women with asthma. Until clinical trials prove that premenstrual asthma is a significant problem, conventional therapy is recommended in the premenstrual state. On the other hand, if a woman has frequent asthma relapses in the premenstrual cycle, asthma medications could be started or stepped up during this period.

Asthma and Pregnancy

One in every ten pregnancies is complicated by asthma. What happens to women with asthma when they become pregnant? The standard answer to this question was one-third get worse, one-third are unchanged, and one-third improve. It is rare or unheard of for labor and delivery to be complicated by acute asthma. Furthermore, most women revert to their pre-pregnancy asthma status within three months after their delivery.

Women with mild asthma usually remain stable during pregnancy, whereas women with more moderate to severe asthma are likely to worsen. These people will need closer observation during pregnancy than those women with mild asthma. As asthma may increase the risk of complications for both the mother and the baby, we must determine the reasons for asthma complications during pregnancy. Poorly controlled asthma may lead to low oxygen levels, elevated blood pressure, and dehydration, all of which adversely affect the mother and developing fetus. Mothers with lower lung function tests have more intrauterine growth retardation, implying that poor asthma control leads to adverse outcomes. Studies that compared asthma in pregnancy managed by asthma specialists versus non-specialists found a lower rate of mortality and low birth weight infants in people who received specialty care.

Risks in Pregnancy

Some of the older medical literature on pregnancy and asthma downplayed the risk asthma poses to the fetus and mother. I no longer tell my pregnant mothers not to worry. Several studies comparing outcomes in mothers with asthma to outcomes in non-asthmatic mothers reported an increase in infant mortality, premature or low birth weight, toxemia of pregnancy, and high blood pressure. The risk of these complications is much higher in asthmatic mothers who smoke, especially African-American women.

Dr. Kitaw Demissie studied nearly five hundred thousand births in several New Jersey hospitals between 1989 and 1992. Demissie identified 2,289 asthmatic mothers and compared their pregnancy outcomes to non-asthmatic mothers. The mothers with asthma had more than a three-fold greater risk of delivering a premature or low-birth-weight infant. Asthmatic mothers were more likely to have preeclampsia or high blood pressure in pregnancy, require a longer hospital stay, and need a cesarean section. The risk for congenital defects was only slightly higher in the mothers with asthma. Asthma control in these New Jersey mothers may have been less than ideal, as most mothers did not receive specialty care during pregnancy.

Asthma specialists believe that when asthma is well controlled in pregnancy, the risk for complications is minimal. This concept is supported by a report from Kaiser-Permanente's Prospective Study of Asthma During Pregnancy. In this study of 486 pregnant asthmatic women actively managed by asthma specialists, there was no increase in the incidence of preeclampsia, perinatal mortality, prematurity, or congenital defects. Upper respiratory tract infections are the most common triggers of severe asthma in pregnancy. The peak incidence of asthma relapses in pregnancy occurs between the twenty-fourth and thirty-sixth week of pregnancy. Asthma usually improves during the last four weeks of pregnancy. One study that needs to be confirmed is a recent survey in Finland that found that infants delivered by cesarean section were at more risk to develop asthma.

In 1993, the National Asthma Education and Prevention Program established the Working Group on Asthma and Pregnancy. Twelve physicians from various specialties recommended the following integrated asthma and obstetric management program:

- Periodic lung function tests to detect early warning signs of relapsing asthma. This can be accomplished by home monitoring with peak flow meters and in-office assessment with spirometry. The group emphasized the need for fetal monitoring, including ultrasound and daily kick counts to evaluate fetal activity.
- Avoidance of asthma triggers is extremely important during pregnancy, as appropriate environmental controls reduce the need for asthma medications and acute care visits for asthma.
- Ongoing allergy injections can be continued in pregnancy, but allergy injections should not be started during pregnancy.
- Stepwise drug therapy with a careful step-up and step-down approach as discussed in the section on asthma guidelines.

The National Asthma Education and Prevention Program enrolled 1,739 pregnant women with asthma who were classified into three categories based on the severity of their disease. Fifty percent were classified as mild, 47 percent had moderate disease, and 3 percent had severe disease. The results of this study were recently published. One-third of all the people in the study got worse in pregnancy, whereas 23 percent improved. The severity of asthma closely predicted who got better and who got worse. In other words, those with more severe asthma at the outset had more problems in pregnancy. Thus, these expectant mothers need more aggressive treatment and closer followup than those with milder asthma.

A Closer Look at Drug Therapy in Pregnancy

The principles of asthma therapy during pregnancy differ very little from the treatment of non-pregnant women. The proper approach combines drug therapy, environmental controls and, when indicated, allergy injections or immunotherapy. There should be no holding back of drugs considered to be safe in pregnancy. The benefits of taking asthma drugs in pregnancy far outweigh the risks of uncontrolled asthma that could endanger the life of the fetus and mother.

What, then, are the best asthma medicines for the pregnant asthmatic? The Food and Drug Administration has divided all drugs into categories A, B, and C, based on their relative level of safety during pregnancy. No asthma medication licensed by the FDA falls in the safest category, A. Several drugs are listed in categories B and C. The National Asthma Education Working Group on Asthma and Pregnancy has published recommendations for preferred medications in pregnancy. The tendency is to use older, more proven medications that have a longer track record than the newer asthma drugs. The Asthma Education Working Group recommended that pregnant and breast-feeding mothers avoid the following drugs:

- Alpha-adrenergic compounds (except pseudoephedrine)
- Epinephrine (except in anaphylaxis)
- Iodides
- Sulfonamides
- Tetracyclines
- Quinolones

Asthma medications preferred for use during pregnancy are the following:

- Inhaled beta-agonists (no specific one was endorsed)
- Terbutaline (when systemic beta-agonist therapy is required)
- Theophylline
- Cromolyn sodium (Intal)
- Vanceril, Beclovent, Q-Var, Pulmicort
- Prednisone or prednisolone

Several new asthma medications, including salmeterol (Serevent), the leukotriene modifiers, and many potent inhaled cortisone drugs, have become available since the Working Group completed its report. There is no solid data in pregnancy on the leukotriene modifiers. Most asthma specialists prefer the shorter-acting, beta-agonist drugs like albuterol during pregnancy.

When an inhaled cortisone drug is needed during pregnancy, the drug of choice is now budesonide (Pulmicort Turbuhaler). In January 2002, data from Sweden prompted the FDA to upgrade the pregnancy rating for budesonide from category C to category B—making it the first cortisone drug to receive this rating. The FDA based this labeling change on data that looked at more than two thousand pregnancies in Sweden from 1995 to 1997 that found no increased risk for congenital malformations when budesonide was administered during early pregnancy—the period when most major organ malformations can occur. This drug is also the only inhaled cortisone drug with a once-a-day dosing indication for children and adults with mild to moderate asthma.

The data on oral cortisone use in pregnancy is not encouraging. Pregnant women who took oral cortisone drugs had more pregnancy complications. Again, it is believed that the complications in pregnancy were due to the severity of the asthma and not the oral cortisone. In cases of severe asthma, the benefit of oral cortisone for the mother and baby far outweighs the risks of severe asthma. While theophylline has generally been considered to be safe in pregnancy, a recent report on asthmatic women who took theophylline throughout pregnancy raises some concerns. Three pregnant women who used theophylline and beta-agonist inhalers delivered children with severe congenital heart defects. Studies in chick embryos have shown that high doses of theophylline can cause congenital heart defects. These findings suggest that theophylline should be avoided in pregnancy.

Obviously, the ideal drug therapy during pregnancy is no therapy, especially during the first three months of pregnancy when the likelihood of fetal malformation is greatest. However, no matter what is done, remember that three to five percent of all pregnant women will deliver an infant with a birth defect and two-thirds of the time the cause of the birth defect is unknown. Several prospective studies are underway to determine the safety of asthma drugs during pregnancy. Many of these studies will be the first to look at pregnancy outcomes on a prospective basis. GlaxoSmithKline has developed a registry program to evaluate the effects of several drugs during pregnancy. Drugs used for common conditions like migraine headaches, antiviral therapy, and anti-epileptic medication will be evaluated. This laudable effort may help to pinpoint those drugs that cause birth defects. The American College of Allergy, Asthma and Immunology has established a registry for pregnant asthmatics to gather more information.

Allergy Testing During Pregnancy

Allergy tests should be postponed until pregnancy is completed. There is a small risk that allergy testing might trigger an allergic reaction which in turn could provoke premature labor. Allergy injections or immunotherapy is safe during pregnancy. One study of 121 pregnancies in 90 women receiving immunotherapy found no increase in perinatal complications in a treated group versus a non-treated control group. It is recommended that allergen immunotherapy be continued during pregnancy in women who have reached a maintenance dose. I recommend a dose reduction to minimize the risk of a systemic reaction. No competent allergist or asthma specialist would recommend starting allergy injections during pregnancy.

The Eight-Step AAFA Asthma Plan

The Asthma and Allergy Foundation of America (AAFA) published the Eight-Step Asthma Plan in 2000 that concisely summarizes the proper approach to asthma in pregnancy.

Step 1: Form a strong team between your primary care provider, asthma specialist, and your obstetrician. Be sure all health-care providers know about your asthma and your pregnancy.

Step 2: Keep taking your asthma medications. Avoid all other medications. Be sure to discuss all medications with your team of doctors or nurses. Know which medications to avoid during pregnancy.

Step 3: Continue your regular allergy shots. Do not start allergy shots or increase doses during pregnancy.

Step 4: Get a flu shot and try to avoid people, especially young children, who have repeated respiratory infections. Frequent hand washing may ward off unwanted viral infections.

Step 5: Aim for good control of your asthma every day. Keep a journal of your peak flow readings and use of asthma medications.

Step 6: Monitor, monitor, monitor! When asthma is unstable, use your peak flow meters daily. Your doctors should also check your breathing capacity on a regular basis with a spirometer, as peak flow readings may not always portray a true picture of your lung functions. Ultrasound and fetal heart rate monitoring will follow your baby's progress.

Step 7: Avoid asthma triggers, irritants, and allergens.

Step 8: Do not smoke and avoid people who do. If you do smoke, make every effort to stop. Remember those infants exposed to passive smoke or born to mothers who smoke have lower birth weights and are three times more likely to die from Sudden Infant Death Syndrome.

Leaders from several agencies, including the FDA, NIH, and the pharmaceutical industry, have held workshops to review the issues of asthma in pregnancy. They summarized the medical literature and asked the question, "How does the course of asthma change during pregnancy?" The one message that came through loud and clear is that mothers with moderate to severe asthma need to be followed at regular intervals during their pregnancy by both their obstetrician and an asthma specialist. People with moderate to severe asthma should undergo fetal ultrasound and fetal heart rate monitoring at appropriate intervals. It is also important that asthma medications be available in the labor and delivery suite. Both the obstetrician and the anesthesiologist should be prepared to treat an asthma relapse.

In summary, the main goals of asthma management during pregnancy should include prevention of asthma episodes that interfere with sleep or normal activity, maintenance of optimal lung function, and avoidance of adverse drug effects, thereby enabling the normal birth of a healthy infant. Educational efforts should emphasize appropriate inhaler technique, recognition of symptoms, signs of relapsing asthma, and teaching people when to seek medical care. Allowing the patient to express her concerns can reduce stress associated with asthma. One must reassure the pregnant mother that outcomes in properly managed asthma are not significantly different from outcomes in non-asthmatic women.

Breastfeeding and Asthma

The concerns of the asthmatic mother do not end with delivery if she decides to breastfeed her baby. Mothers with allergic asthma should be encouraged to breastfeed, as breastfed infants are less likely to develop eczema, food allergy, or asthma in infancy and early childhood. Even though 10 percent of any drug she takes ends up in her breast milk and is ingested by her baby, there is usually little or no risk to the feeding infant.

One drug that may be troublesome in breastfed infants is oral theophylline. Small amounts of theophylline transferred by breast milk may cause the infant to become irritable or jittery. When such irritability persists, the mother should stop taking theophylline. Inhaled beta-agonist and cortisone drugs have been a boon to nursing mothers, as only trace amounts of these inhaled drugs end up in the mother's breast milk. Nursing mothers who require oral cortisone (prednisone) on a daily or alternate-day basis to control severe asthma should not breastfeed.

Does breastfeeding prevent the development of eczema, food allergies, or asthma? There are conflicting responses to this important question. Controlled trials of breastfeeding can be criticized for a variety of reasons, including inadequate duration of breastfeeding, lack of environmental controls or maternal diet, small sample size, and early introduction of solid foods. The theoretical benefits of breast milk derive from the transfer of maternal antibody that protects the infant from bacterial and viral illnesses. More importantly, breastfed infants avoid the ingestion of sensitizing foods like eggs or cow's milk. A *British Medical Journal* report urged pregnant women with a family history of asthma or allergic disorders like hay fever and eczema to avoid eating peanut products during pregnancy or while breastfeeding. Ingestion of such foods during pregnancy or while breastfeeding may sensitize the fetus or newborn to peanut allergen. I recommend that infants who have eczema, egg or milk allergy, asthma, or a strong family history of allergy avoid peanut and tree nut products until their third birthday. The American Academy of Pediatrics now recommends that all "at risk infants," (positive family history of allergy, especially on the mother's side), avoid milk products until age one, egg products until age two, and tree nuts/peanuts and seafood until age three.

Older data suggests that breastfeeding forestalls but does not prevent the onset of asthma or allergic diseases later on in childhood. Newer studies suggest breastfeeding may be permanently protective. Dr. Wendy Oddy believes breastfeeding for four months may prevent childhood asthma. Oddy followed 2,187 Australian children from birth to age six and found that infants who were breastfed for more than four months were less likely to have asthma at age six. Oddy speculated that breastfeeding might modify the immune system and divert it down the non-allergy-asthma Th1 pathway. A long-term study of children in Tucson, Arizona, found that breastfeeding protected against asthma, but only in those infants who had no other allergic problems. The duration of breastfeeding may be critical. It may be more protective when prolonged for six months. In China, where there is a very low incidence of asthma, infants may be breastfed for three years or longer. Thus, until additional studies are completed, the questions revolving around the protective effects of breastfeeding remain unresolved. In my opinion the scale tips in the direction of protection from asthma and other allergic diseases. Thus, when given the opportunity, I strongly advise all pregnant mothers to breastfeed for at least six months, especially if there is a strong family history of asthma or other allergic diseases. When high risk infants cannot be breastfed, I recommend consulting with your pediatrician about feeding infants with non-soy, non-milk, or hydrolysate formulas.

CHAPTER TWENTY-ONE

Adult Asthma

While most victims of asthma develop the disease in early childhood, many people start to wheeze in adulthood for the first time in their lives. This form of asthma is called adult-onset asthma. When I first encounter a new patient with adult-onset asthma, I closely question them about their health in childhood. At first, many deny having any asthma during childhood, but on closer questioning they often recall being allergic or "bronchial" during their childhood. To me this suggests that they had undiagnosed childhood asthma that went into remission for several years. Another important variable to look at in adult-onset asthma is the history of exposure to environmental tobacco smoke. Adults with bronchitis or chronic lung disease due to exposure to environmental tobacco smoke are often mislabeled as having asthma.

Adult-Onset Asthma

Adult-onset asthma is quite different from childhood asthma. There is often no association with family history, hay fever, eczema, or food allergies. The typical case of adult-onset asthma in a nonsmoker often begins with a simple respiratory infection that becomes a bronchitis-like illness that never clears up. Coughing and wheezing may persist for weeks, months, and sometimes years before the diagnosis of asthma is entertained. This type of "post-infectious asthma" is the least understood of all forms of asthma.

When I first started to practice, I thought that adults with adult-onset asthma got better with age. After following hundreds of these patients for nearly thirty years, I know that this is not the case. Only one in every five people with adult-onset asthma experiences a significant remission. Adult-onset asthma is usually more severe and less reversible than childhood-onset asthma, especially in women who start wheezing after age fifty. Many people with adult-onset asthma experience a severe and rapid decline in lung function. Asthmatics who smoke have the most severe decline in lung function. Most studies on the prognosis or long-term outlook of asthma have focused on children and young adults. An Italian study of 18,000 adults found that late-onset asthma was less likely to go into remission. There is little solid data looking at the prognosis of adult-onset asthma. One reason that the clinical course of adult-onset asthma is so unclear is that it is often confused with chronic bronchitis or emphysema.

Doctor Charles Reed reviewed the records of 242 Mayo Clinic asthmatics over age sixty-five. Reed found that the majority of elderly people with asthma had severe airway obstruction and many of these people had had asthma for only a short period of time. In contrast, people with a history of childhood asthma had better lung function and less severe disease. Adults with positive skin tests and an allergic component to their asthma had milder asthma than those people with negative skin tests (so-called intrinsic asthma). Obviously, elderly asthmatics who smoke or have previously smoked have more severe asthma. Or it may be that adult-onset asthma is more likely to cause airway remodeling, where the bronchial tubes are permanently damaged and scarred. This select group of severe adult-onset asthmatics often requires aggressive and persistent use of all classes of asthma drugs. Many will require an oral cortisone drug to bring their asthma under control when their lung functions do not improve. More studies are needed to unravel the mysteries of adult-onset asthma.

One new and very disturbing finding in adults with asthma is that sufferers may be more prone to heart disease. Kaiser-Permanente investigators in California studied the medical records of 1,062 non-smoking asthmatics. They found that active asthmatics were 32 percent more likely to have heart disease. The reason for the higher risk of heart disease in these people is unclear. It is possible that the inflammation in the asthmatic lung might also occur in the coronary arteries.

Asthma in the Elderly

The number of individuals over age sixty-five is rapidly increasing worldwide. Senior citizens, who now account for one in every eight Americans, represent the fastest-growing segment of developed societies. Health surveys find that the rate of asthma is rising in this population. Nearly 2 million American senior citizens have asthma and another million probably have undiagnosed asthma. Elderly individuals who develop asthma are more likely to suffer from nasal polyps, sinus problems, and gastroesophageal reflux disease (GERD). Like many other diseases, asthma in the elderly is often overlooked. This is ironic, as the prevalence of asthma in the United States is higher among the elderly than in all other age groups except children under age eighteen. Older women are more likely to develop late-onset adult asthma, suggesting that postmenopausal hormonal changes associated with aging may play a role in adult-onset asthma.

Asthma is widely under-diagnosed in the elderly. Physicians often label a coughing and wheezing senior citizen as having chronic bronchitis or emphysema. Undiagnosed asthma may explain why the death rate for asthma in the elderly is ten times that of younger asthmatics. Dr. Paul Enright discovered a large number of senior citizens with undiagnosed asthma in an ongoing Cardiovascular Health Study at the University of Arizona. Four in every ten of these people were not using any asthma medication whatsoever. Enright's study points out the need to improve the rate of asthma diagnosis in the elderly, and dispels the myth that asthma is a disease that rarely starts later on in life.

There are several reasons why asthma is under-diagnosed in the elderly. Physiologic changes associated with aging that can mask the presence of asthma include low lung functions, decreased mucus production, and an ineffective cough mechanism. Many senior citizens feel that coughing, wheezing, or shortness of breath is just part of getting old. Coexisting depression may disguise an underlying chronic disease like asthma. Another consideration is that many elderly asthmatics are "poor perceivers" of asthma. This means they do not feel any shortness of breath or chest discomfort until their lung functions are way below normal. These poor perceivers have an increased risk of fatal or near-fatal asthma due to the fact that they cannot detect mild airway obstruction. They seek treatment only when airflow obstruction is far advanced. This concept was supported by a study of survivors of near-fatal asthma, who were found to have an impaired ability to detect bronchoconstriction. Following lung function with peak flow meters becomes even more important when treating poor perceivers with asthma. Laboratory studies in the elderly should include full lung function tests, a total eosinophil count, and an allergic antibody or serum IgE test.

Should elderly asthmatics undergo allergy skin testing? I used to believe that skin testing was not always indicated in elderly asthmatics as previous studies found that only 20 percent of elderly people with asthma had positive skin tests to aeroallergens. This picture is changing—even the elderly are becoming more allergic. Dr. Richard Huss of Johns Hopkins recently looked at eighty elderly people with persistent asthma and found that nearly 75 percent tested positive to at least one aeroallergen. Cat was the most prevalent positive skin test, and

Bermuda grass was the second most common. More than half of these people were exposed to significant levels of dust mites and 30 percent were exposed to cockroach allergen. Nearly two-thirds had moderate to severe asthma. Yet, only two-thirds were taking inhaled cortisone drugs. Huss's study stresses the importance of diagnostic allergy skin testing in elderly asthmatics. In my recent experience, a surprising number of elderly people have unrecognized dust mite, mold, or animal allergy. Thus, in my opinion, allergy skin testing is definitely indicated in all elderly people with asthma.

Asthma Management in the Elderly

Elderly asthmatics experience significant relief and improvement in symptoms and lung functions with proper asthma treatment. Due to coexisting diseases and complicated drug programs, asthma management in this age group becomes more complex. Asthma therapy in the elderly should focus on the individual's mental and physical capacity. Many people will require a polypharmacy, or multiple drug, approach that includes the short-acting and long-acting beta-agonists, inhaled cortisone medications, the leukotriene modifiers, or theophylline. A few elderly asthmatics will require oral cortisone drugs. Medication errors and misunderstanding of the use of medications are common in the elderly. The high costs of asthma medications and lack of insurance coverage may force elderly asthmatics to cut back on their medications or resort to less effective and more dangerous over-the-counter (OTC) medications.

Drug interactions are more of a problem in this age group, as many of these people take additional medications for other chronic diseases like high blood pressure or heart disease. The use of metered dose inhalers is a challenge for this group, as studies have shown that only one in three elderly asthmatics correctly use their inhalers. Certain devices that can help the elderly patient to follow an asthma treatment plan include color-coded medications, daily charts, calendars, and pillboxes. It is imperative that these people receive close supervision and instruction in the use of inhalers and spacing devices. Nebulizers are a great help in administering medications when people have trouble using metered dose inhalers. It is best to instruct senior citizens on a one-on-one basis and provide a written asthma action plan at each visit. I try to find a family member, neighbor, or friend to periodically check on compliance with medication programs if an elderly patient lives alone. In some instances it is necessary to request a home visit from the local Visiting Nurse Association or an asthma educator.

Drug Interactions

Decreased kidney and liver function associated with aging can lead to difficulty in metabolizing asthma drugs. Common side effects and drug interactions encountered in elderly asthmatics are listed below:

- High doses of inhaled beta-agonists may lower serum potassium levels, especially in people who are taking prednisone or fluid pills. Low potassium symptoms like muscle cramps are best treated by taking extra potassium in the form of bananas, orange juice, or potassium pills.
- Elderly asthmatics are more prone to easy bruising after taking oral or inhaled cortisone drugs. Oral cortisone drugs may also increase blood pressure.
- It is best to use the closed-mouth technique when using inhaler drugs like Atrovent and Combivent as these drugs may aggravate glaucoma if accidentally sprayed into the eye.
- Senior citizens are more likely to experience adverse reactions to antihistamines, including dry mouth, dizziness, bladder or prostate problems, and sedation. These reactions are minimized with the new non-sedating antihistamines.
- The use of beta-blocking drugs for glaucoma, high blood pressure, and heart disease can aggravate asthma.

• Theophylline drugs lower the pressure between the esophagus and stomach, thereby aggravating gastroesophageal reflux disease (GERD).

Elderly asthmatics should be encouraged to exercise. In my experience, one of the best forms of exercise in this age group is swimming. Many of my elderly patients have shown unbelievable improvement in their lung functions after joining an aerobic or active swimming program. Calcium and vitamin D help combat osteoporosis. As the need for emergency or elective surgery is more likely in elderly people, careful preoperative evaluation is necessary. Health-care providers must be sure that both the surgeon and anesthesiologist are aware of the patient's asthma and asthma drug program. All elderly asthmatics should receive an annual flu shot and the pneumonia vaccine, Pneumovax.

CHAPTER TWENTY-TWO

Step-Up Versus Step-Down Therapy

Some people need to start high and then step down, while others benefit from starting low and then stepping up. The newly diagnosed patient with mild persistent asthma does not usually need to start with a higher dose of an inhaled anti-inflammatory drug, as they can be easily controlled with low or moderate doses. On the other hand, people showing more moderate to severe asthma will require the more aggressive step-down approach. I will often start these patients on a short course of oral cortisone and higher doses of long-term-controlling medications in an effort to normalize lung functions. People with poor asthma control (nighttime wheezing, need for more rescue medications, or urgent care visits) require step-up therapy. Step-up therapy may include doubling the dose of an inhaled cortisone drug, starting a short-term pulse of prednisone, or adding other long-term-controlling medications like the beta-agonists and the leukotriene modifiers.

While the NHLBI Guidelines precisely outline the use of asthma medicines when the patient is coughing and wheezing, they do not tell the asthma caregiver how to fine-tune asthma medications. Once patients have stabilized, I will fine-tune or step down medications to the lowest possible dose that controls asthma. In general the last medication added can be the first to be reduced or eliminated. In other words—"last in, first out." At certain times of the year, particularly during a change of season, people with asthma may require asthma medications on a daily basis, whereas at other times of the year—often mid-summer or mid-winter—some people can revert to an as-needed schedule. These decisions are more difficult for people with moderate asthma, whose needs can vary from day to day, week to week, season to season, and year to year.

My personal approach to patients with persistent asthma who have varying needs for medications is as follows: If they are taking their asthma medications on a regular basis, say two times a day, I tell them to taper to once a day when they have been symptom-free or have normal peak flow readings for two to three months. If they are symptom-free for another month or so, they may be able to stop their medications completely and revert to an as-needed schedule.

If your asthma recurs or peak flow readings fall while tapering medicines, you might be instructed to revert to the previous medication schedule that controlled asthma symptoms or kept your peak flow readings at normal levels. When you get a chest cold or a respiratory infection, you should resume or increase your medications. In essence, I try to instruct the patients (or parents) to be their own asthma doctor. People with asthma are taught to contact their primary physician or my office in the early stages of an asthma relapse that may require antibiotics or prednisone. Not every patient or family can be handled in this manner, as self-management requires a certain level of patient motivation, judgment, asthma education, and intelligence.

One recent study implied that doctors may be prescribing too much inhaled cortisone to their asthma patients. This study looked at eight asthma studies in 2,324 people with asthma and found that 80 percent of the benefit achieved at higher doses of an inhaled cortisone drug could be obtained at much lower doses. In other words, a low dose may work just as well as a higher dose in most people. This finding makes it even more imperative to constantly adjust asthma sufferers to the lowest possible dose of inhaled cortisone.

Pediatric Guidelines

The approach to managing asthma in children under the age of five is really no different than older children and adults. Nevertheless, separate guidelines for pediatric asthma, entitled *Pediatric Asthma: Promoting Best Practice,* were published in late 1999. These are the first set of asthma guidelines devoted entirely to the pediatric patient. The goal of this publication is to ensure that health-care providers who manage pediatric asthma learn about, understand, and implement clinical and best-practice information for diagnosing and managing children with asthma. These well-referenced, user-friendly guidelines can be obtained from AAAAI or via the AAAAI Web site at http://www.aaaai.org

Treat Early and Often?

One of the dilemmas faced by doctors treating newly diagnosed asthma in young children is deciding when to start an inhaled cortisone drug. Published guidelines for young children urged the use of non-cortisone medications such as cromolyn or Intal. While this approach usually works well in children with milder asthma, it does not always control patients with moderate or severe persistent asthma. You would have to take Intal three to four times a day, and it often takes weeks for Intal to take effect. This approach may not be the best way to treat early-onset childhood asthma. In the past few years, asthma specialists have learned that most of the deterioration in lung function that occurs in young asthmatic children occurs by age seven. Thus, one must ask a very important question. Would the early use of inhaled cortisone drugs in young children optimize lung function and prevent permanent lung damage? Let me explain why my answer to this question is yes—treat early and often.

Doctor Terri Haahtela from Helsinki, Finland, studied 103 newly diagnosed children with asthma over a two-year period. These children were assigned to two treatment groups. One group received the inhaled cortisone drug, budesonide (Pulmicort), twice a day. The other group only took an inhaled beta-agonist, terbutaline (Brethine), on an as-needed basis. After two years, children on budesonide (Pulmicort) had better peak flow rates and symptom scores, and fewer asthma relapses. This study concluded that early use of inhaled cortisone resulted in greater improvement than the as-needed use of a rescue bronchodilator. This (and other) studies have convinced me that the early use of an inhaled cortisone drug in young asthmatic children may prevent permanent lung damage later on in life.

There is no doubt that children with persistent asthma have chronic inflammation in their bronchial tubes. Likewise, there is no question that treatment with inhaled cortisone reduces or even reverses this inflammation. Thus, early intervention with inhaled cortisone drugs is becoming the treatment of choice in these young children with persistent asthma. Since inhaled cortisone drugs have only been available for a little more than two decades, there are no long-term studies that tell us if early use of inhaled cortisone in a four-year-old child will prevent permanent lung disease when this child reaches age fifty or sixty. Some proponents of the leukotriene modifiers suggest that these drugs can take the place of the inhaled cortisone drugs in mild persistent asthma. Evolving studies will eventually answer this important question. At the present time, I prefer to use an inhaled cortisone drug in all forms of persistent asthma.

How important is it to diagnose persistent asthma early in the course of the disease? Unfortunately, it is very difficult to pick out those infants and children who are at risk of developing irreversible lung damage or remodeling. I believe early diagnosis and aggressive treatment may vastly improve one's chances of being wheeze-free later on in life. Let me further explain why there may be a window of opportunity in early childhood asthma where treatment with an inhaled cortisone drug may lead to a permanent asthma remission in adolescence or adulthood.

In my early years of practice in the 1970s, the pre–inhaled cortisone drug era, I treated scores of children and young adults with severe asthma. As inhaled cortisone drugs were not yet available, many of these people only managed their asthma when they took oral prednisone on a daily or alternate-day basis. When I received a phone call from one of these patients or their parents during the evening or on a weekend, I knew that I was in for a long ordeal. Many of these patients had labile asthma that could quickly develop into severe, life-threatening asthma, which would require immediate hospitalization and treatment in an intensive care unit. Despite the dramatic increase in the incidence of asthma and the size of my practice since that time, I do not encounter this type of patient nearly as often as I did in the pre–inhaled cortisone era. Presently, none of my child or young adult patients with persistent asthma require alternate-day prednisone. In my opinion the main reason for this change in asthma severity is the availability and early use of inhaled cortisone drugs in childhood.

I see patients of all ages with asthma. Over the past ten years I have been impressed with a drop-off in the number of young adults in their twenties and thirties who have severe asthma and poor lung functions. Most young asthmatic adults have mild impairment in their lung functions and show no evidence of permanent lung damage, as opposed to my older adult patients who often have poor lung functions. Although I am seeing more young and middle-aged adults with asthma, they are not as severely impaired as older, non-smoking asthmatics in their fifties and sixties. I believe the decline in severe asthma in young adults is due to the fact that they took inhaled cortisone drugs in their childhood, whereas these inhaled cortisone drugs were not available to the older generation of asthmatics. In my opinion, early introduction of inhaled cortisone prevents remodeling and scarring or the bronchial tubes.

How Long Treatment Lasts

Most people respond to an inhaled cortisone drug within days or weeks. In moderate to more severe asthma three to nine months of treatment may be required to show major improvement. Some people require more than one year of treatment before reaching a full response. Abrupt withdrawal of a cortisone inhaler may evoke a recurrence of symptoms, usually within a month. Regular inhaled cortisone therapy, once started, will usually continue indefinitely, unless a causative agent in the workplace can be identified and avoided. When prescribed inhaled cortisone, some people ask, "How long will I or my child have to take this drug?" A Netherlands study looked at the effects of stopping inhaled cortisone in a group of children who had been using these drugs for nearly three years. They found that when the inhaled cortisone drug was stopped, most children rapidly relapsed to the level of asthma they had before the drug was started. Thus, the message is that inhaled cortisone drugs do not cure asthma, and long-term treatment may be necessary in people with moderate to severe asthma.

Take a Deep Breath: Lung Function Tests

One final important point needs to be made regarding the asthma guidelines. Both adult and pediatric guidelines emphatically state that spirometry or lung function testing is the "gold standard of asthma diagnosis and management." Spirometry is recommended at the initial visit, after starting treatment, and at least once a year after that to properly evaluate the effectiveness of asthma therapy. I wish to emphasize this critical point. In my experience, most primary health-care providers are not using spirometers in their office or clinic. Due to convenience and cost constraints, many health-care providers rely on the less expensive peak flow meters. In my opinion, relying on peak flow meters alone to assess the status of moderate to severe asthma can lead to serious errors in asthma management. I have seen scores of patients with unstable asthma who blow normal readings on their peak flow meter but have lung function or spirometry tests that are markedly abnormal. Any health-care provider who treats moderate or severe persistent asthma on a regular basis should monitor their patients' lung functions with a spirometer.

Acute Asthma

Prior to 1990, most people with acute asthma attacks were sent to emergency rooms where oxygen and X-ray facilities were available, and where blood theophylline levels and arterial blood gases could be done to assess the severity of the acute asthma attack. Now many people come to their physician's office or clinic for treatment of acute asthma. There are valid reasons for this emerging trend. First, chest X-rays and blood gas studies are not needed in most cases of acute asthma. Second, acute asthma care is undoubtedly more cost-effective in a clinic or office setting. The majority of people with acute asthma are not that seriously ill, even though many people have been wheezing for several days or weeks before they contact their health-care provider. While modern-day emergency room physicians have the expertise and experience to competently resolve an acute asthma episode, they may not have the time to implement the asthma education programs that prevent future asthma relapses. When first evaluating an acute asthma attack in the doctor's office or clinic, it is important to assess the severity of the attack. Danger signals during an acute episode include the following:

• Severe coughing and wheezing
• Using neck and rib muscles to breathe
• Chest tightness
• Inability to talk
• Cyanosis (discoloration of lips and fingernails)

The quickest way to objectively assess the severity of an attack is to measure oxygen levels, as well as lung function or peak flow rates.

People with severe wheezing, cyanosis (discoloration of lips and fingernails), an inability to talk, or a previous history of life-threatening asthma should always be referred to a fully equipped emergency room. Severe asthma setbacks can be minimized or prevented when asthma sufferers and their families learn the ten early warning signs of deteriorating asthma:

1. Excessive absence from school or work
2. Cough and wheezing unresponsive to medications
3. Wheezing with minimal exertion
4. Need for inhaler every two or three hours
5. Constant wheezing during sleep
6. Persistent high fever
7. Severe neck or chest pain
8. Persistent vomiting
9. Difficulty speaking because of wheezing
10. Cyanosis (discoloration of lips and fingernails)

The presence of one or more of these ten early warning signs is a clear-cut sign that this "out-of-control asthma" requires immediate medical attention from a primary-care doctor, or emergency room or asthma specialist. Additional risk factors that mandate immediate care in relapsing asthma are as follows:

- A prior history of near-fatal asthma
- A recent asthma hospitalization
- Repeated emergency room visits
- Chronic use of prednisone
- Recent withdrawal from prednisone
- A past history of fainting or seizures
- Serious psychosocial problems

Acute Asthma Treatment

When an acutely ill patient is initially seen in the office or clinic, the doctor should quickly evaluate the severity of the asthma episode by noting the patient's overall appearance, listening to the chest, and performing an oxygen level and breathing test. The doctor will order an inhalation treatment with a beta-agonist drug. Fortunately, the time-honored practice of administering repeated injections of epinephrine has given way to the more judicious modern-day nebulization or inhalation therapy with short-acting beta-agonists like albuterol or levalbuterol (Xopenex). People no longer have to endure the pallor, tremors, rapid heart rates, and vomiting often associated with epinephrine injections. I usually find it necessary to administer a prednisone pulse in acute asthma. I give the first day's dose in the office to avoid any delay in starting prednisone. People need to be constantly reminded that proper use of their peak flow meter at home may enable them to detect an asthma relapse in its early stages and prevent a sick call or emergency room visit. Several home management techniques shown to be ineffective in acute asthma include drinking large volumes of liquid, breathing moist air or mist from a hot shower, breathing into a bag, and taking over-the-counter antihistamine or cold remedies.

There are three possible responses to the treatment of acute asthma with a beta-agonist—good, fair, and poor. A good response is typified by mild coughing and wheezing, no use of neck or rib muscles, no symptoms at rest, and the ability to climb one flight of stairs. Lung function or peak flow rates are usually 70 percent or better of baseline. A fair or incomplete response after one hour of treatment is characterized by persistent coughing and wheezing. The patient is usually alert with no cyanosis, and minimal use of neck and rib muscles to breathe. This patient may have some symptoms at rest and cannot exercise vigorously. Lung function and peak flow rates are usually between 60 and 70 percent of baseline. At this point, physicians should start a pulse of prednisone. A poor response to inhaled beta-agonist means just that; severe coughing and wheezing persist, you would need to use your rib and neck muscles to breathe, you would not be able speak without gasping, and you would have cyanosis of your lips and nails. Lung function and peak flow rates are usually less than 50 percent of baseline. These are the asthmatics that can and do die from asthma, especially when they delay seeking emergency care. Those patients who do not respond to routine office treatment should be referred to an emergency room where they may be given more inhalation treatments along with an intravenous cortisone drug. If emergency room care does not break the asthma attack, the patient will be admitted to the hospital for additional treatment. The six telltale signs that signal the need for an asthma hospitalization are the following:

- Fast heart rate and rapid respiration
- Using the neck and rib muscles to breathe
- Severe wheezing or inability to speak
- Persistent sweating
- Cyanosis of lips and fingernails
- A disturbed or confused mental state

While children and young adults are more prone to acute asthma episodes, they are also more likely to respond promptly to treatment and avoid hospitalization. Adult asthmatics coming to an emergency room with acute asthma are a different story. They can be very difficult to treat, as adults are more likely to have put off calling their doctor and seeking care. Delays in seeking care make it harder for emergency room physicians to reverse the asthma relapse. As emergency room docs are fond of saying, "The time to treat your acute asthma relapse and prevent you from being hospitalized was yesterday." When you require a hospital stay, doctors use the term "status asthmaticus" to describe your medical condition. Once hospitalized, you would be given oxygen, inhalation therapy, and intravenous cortisone drugs. Most hospitalized asthmatics improve within twenty-four to forty-eight hours.

Acute Respiratory Failure

A small percentage of people who do not respond to in-hospital treatment develop a life-threatening condition called status asthmaticus or acute respiratory failure. In respiratory failure, the bronchial tubes are almost totally blocked. The lungs are deprived of life-sustaining oxygen and cannot eliminate the body's toxic waste gas, carbon dioxide. Picture it as a form of very slow suffocation. Machines must now take over the control of breathing. These people are connected to a breathing machine called a ventilator. A tube is inserted into the trachea or windpipe and the respiratory muscles are deliberately paralyzed. Dials on the machine are then adjusted to deliver the proper amounts of oxygen and remove carbon dioxide. This procedure, called assisted ventilation, may continue for several days. Once the ventilated patient improves, the machine is gradually turned down, and the patient is slowly weaned from the ventilator. Thanks to the development of intensive care units devoted to respiratory care and the ready availability of critical-care doctors, assisted ventilation now has a very low complication and mortality rate. An inpatient asthma death is a very rare event in well-staffed hospitals.

Most asthma deaths now occur suddenly and unexpectedly outside of the hospital. It is my impression, and that of my pulmonary colleagues, that the overall incidence of acute respiratory failure is decreasing. Our practice used to see several asthmatic patients a year who ended up on a ventilator. Now, far fewer patients require this type of intensive treatment. More aggressive use of inhaled cortisone drugs and prompt intervention with prednisone in the early stages of relapsing asthma may be the main reasons for the decline in status asthmaticus.

The Asthma Action Plan

Our practice will often write out an asthma action plan for our asthma patients (Figure 22.1). This written plan is available to the patient, family, primary physicians, school nurses, and emergency room personnel who may be involved in the care of the patient. The purpose of such a plan is to make everyone involved with the patient aware of the severity of the patient's asthma and convey the need for immediate and appropriate care should the patient suffer an asthma relapse. While it may not be necessary to carry this plan with you at all times, it should be used when traveling or visiting medical facilities unfamiliar with your asthma treatment program.

FIGURE 22.1—Treatment of Asthma Based on Severity

	Daily Long-Term Control	Quick Relief
Mild Intermittent • Symptoms 1–2 times/week • Nocturnal symptoms <2 times/month • Exacerbations brief • PFTs ≥ 80% predicted	None	Short-acting bronchodilator
Mild Persistent • Symptoms >2 times/week • Nocturnal symptoms >2 times/month • PFTs ≥ 80% predicted	Anti-inflammatory agent (low-dose inhaled corticosteroid or cromolyn or nedocromil) Alternatives: sustained-release theophylline or leukotriene modifier* for patients ≥ 6 yrs. old	Short-acting bronchodilator
Moderate Persistent • Daily symptoms • Nocturnal symptoms >1 time/week • Exacerbations ≥ 2 times/week; may last days • PFTs >60% and <80% predicted	Anti-inflammatory agent (low-/medium-dose inhaled corticosteroid) plus long-acting bronchodilator (inhaled beta 2-agonist, sustained-release theophylline, or oral long-acting beta 2-agonist); if needed, add medium-/high-dose inhaled corticosteroid and long-acting bronchodilator	Short-acting bronchodilator
Severe Persistent • Continual symptoms • Frequent nocturnal symptoms • Frequent exacerbations • PFTs <60% predicted	Anti-inflammatory agent (high-dose inhaled corticosteroid) and long-acting bronchodilator (inhaled beta 2-agonist, sustained-release theophylline, or oral long-acting beta 2-agonist) and corticosteroid tablets or syrup	Short-acting bronchodilator

PFTs = Pulmonary Function Tests
* The role of leukotriene modifiers in the management of asthma has yet to be fully defined.

CHAPTER TWENTY-THREE

The Asthma Alarm

Even though asthma deaths are on the rise, they are very rare when one considers that millions of children and adults have asthma. Approximately two hundred American children die from asthma each year, yet nearly 6 million children have asthma. This makes the odds of dying from childhood asthma about 30,000 to 1. The odds of dying from adult asthma are quite a bit higher, about 2,000 to 1. The reason I am discussing asthma deaths in detail is not to frighten the reader, but to point out that many, if not most, asthma deaths are totally preventable. I believe the most common cause of an asthma death in children and adults is a failure by the patient or family to recognize the severity of a serious asthma attack. Doctors at the Aberdeen Royal Infirmary in Scotland found that most asthmatics who died had a very poor understanding of their asthma. These people failed to recognize the danger signs of deteriorating asthma, and delayed seeking care until they were critically ill. Studies at the Royal Hospital for Sick Children in Bristol, England, found that most of the children who died from asthma did so in the middle of the night before they reached the hospital. Tragically, the parents of these children failed to recognize the severity of the nocturnal attack, and many did not want to bother their family doctor in the middle of the night. Unlike other asthma death studies, the Bristol report did not find that asthma deaths were sudden and totally unexpected. In most cases, there was ample time to treat and save the child. The high risk of nocturnal asthma has been identified in subsequent studies. Seventy percent of all near-fatal and fatal asthma attacks occur between midnight and 8:00 a.m.

In an attempt to identify patient profiles and triggers of near-fatal and fatal asthma, I conducted a survey of asthma specialists to gather case reports and analyze the characteristics of people experiencing

RISK FACTORS FOR NEAR-FATAL AND FATAL ASTHMA

In 1985, Doctors Robert Strunk and David Mrazek, from Denver's National Jewish Hospital, reviewed the medical records of twenty-one people who died after they were discharged from this world-renowned asthma center and compared them to a similar number of survivors. The profiles of the survivors were quite different from those who died from asthma. The people who died were more likely to have severe psychological problems not found in the surviving group. As a result of their study, Strunk and Mrazek developed the following profile of the high-risk patient with asthma:

- A history of seizures associated with asthma
- A recent decrease in prednisone doses
- Wheezing at the time of hospital discharge
- A disregard of wheezing and other symptoms
- Poor self-care while in the hospital
- Conflicts with staff and parents
- Use of asthma to manipulate people
- Emotional disturbance and depression
- Severe family disruption

near-fatal and fatal asthma. A questionnaire was distributed to four hundred asthma specialists, most of whom practiced in New England. Near-fatal asthma was defined as asthma requiring out-of-hospital CPR, on-site or in-hospital intubation (putting in a breathing tube), and mechanical ventilation (using a respirator). Characteristics assessed in the survey included age, sex, race, duration of asthma, severity of asthma, lability or brittleness of asthma (history of wide swings in peak flow rates or lung function tests), and existence of other allergic diseases like allergic rhinitis, eczema, and food or drug allergy.

This survey gathered twenty-five reports of near-fatal asthma and twenty cases of fatal asthma. The average age of those experiencing fatal asthma (twenty-two years old) was younger than that of the survivors of a near-fatal event (thirty years old).

Survey Findings

My survey supports the disturbing observation that younger allergic people experience life-threatening asthma suddenly and unexpectedly outside the hospital, as only two near-fatal episodes and one fatal event took place in a hospital setting. Most of these people nearly died or died suddenly and unexpectedly at home, en route to the hospital, in physicians' offices, or in public places such as county fairs, automobiles, and schools. Clinical triggers for near-fatal and fatal asthma included respiratory infections and ingested, inhaled, or injected allergens. Two people succumbed to peanut or tree nut ingestion. Four people experienced near-fatal or fatal asthma after exercising in cold winter weather. Two people who died after running in colder weather might have over-relied on their home nebulizer and delayed seeking appropriate emergency room care. One patient died at home while setting up a home nebulizer for an inhalation treatment. The tragic sequence of over-relying on home nebulizers has previously been cited as a risk factor in both near-fatal and fatal asthma. The risk factor for near-fatal and fatal asthma posed by exercising in colder weather has been infrequently noted. All subjects in both groups were using a short-acting, inhaled beta-agonist drug, and 20 percent of near-fatal and fatal victims were reportedly using a long-acting beta-agonist. Beta-agonist abuse was cited as a contributing factor in four people with near-fatal asthma and nine with fatal asthma. Unlike other studies, where under-utilization of inhaled cortisone drugs is commonly noted in life-threatening asthma, the majority of people in both groups were reportedly using an inhaled cortisone drug. Most of these people had unstable asthma, characterized by wide swings in their lung function tests. This observation is in agreement with other reports that noted that people with severe bronchial hyperreactivity and blunted perception of the severity of their attack were more prone to life-threatening attacks of asthma.

While approximately 50 percent of the people in this survey were thought to have poor compliance and severe disease affected by adverse psychosocial problems, good to excellent compliance was noted in half of those people experiencing near-fatal asthma and fatal episodes. Three patients died on long holiday weekends, where a delay in seeking care may have been a factor. This observation of an increase in near-fatal and fatal episodes on weekends, especially on Sundays, has previously been reported. In one study, 40 percent of asthma deaths took place between Friday night and Monday morning.

Nearly half of the collected cases occurred suddenly and unexpectedly in young, allergic, and compliant asthmatics who did not have a severe high-risk asthma profile. Tragically, several people in this survey might not have died had they not exercised in colder weather, over-relied on their home nebulizer, inadvertently ingested nuts or peanuts, or delayed seeking medical care on holiday weekends.

CHAPTER TWENTY-FOUR

The Psychological Factors in Asthma

Today there is no doubt that asthma is an immunologically driven disease. Yet, asthma specialists agree that psychological factors can be important in many people with asthma. Moderate to severe asthma leads to stress and emotional strain, which then sets up a vicious cycle of worsening asthma. Asthma sufferers should be aware that a wide range of emotions, including crying or even laughing, may trigger asthma. After the introduction of more effective asthma therapies in the 1980s, interest in the psychological aspects of asthma waned. However, the emerging asthma epidemic has rekindled awareness of this topic.

Many people with moderate to severe asthma deny their symptoms and knowingly expose themselves to asthma triggers. Doctor Robert Strunk has found that obese asthmatic children are more likely to have severe psychological problems. He has outlined a psychological profile for high-risk asthma. High-risk asthma sufferers have severe psychological dysfunction, chronic depression, and problems interacting with their medical providers and peers.

The most important form of psychological therapy in these situations is family therapy. Family therapy and asthma self-help programs will help you learn more about asthma mechanisms, triggers, warning signs, and drug management. Some of the themes addressed include poor communication patterns, fear of death, denial of disease, and non-compliance on the part of the patient or family.

How the Average Family Copes

What are the effects of asthma on the average family with an asthmatic child? The National Jewish Hospital in Denver, Colorado, surveyed several hundred patients and families affected by asthma. These families averaged ten office visits per year. Afflicted children averaged eight to fifteen lost school days per year. Half of the parents reported that asthma caused depression in their children, and four of ten parents felt that their child was overly concerned about becoming ill. One-third experienced guilt feelings after an asthma attack. Strained relationships were common between family members and directly correlated with the severity of the asthma.

The Effect of Stress on Asthma

Stress can be defined as environmental demands that tax or exceed a person's ability to cope, resulting in both psychological and biological changes that place the person at risk for disease. Stress stimulates the nervous system and triggers asthma through multiple mechanisms. Children exposed to inner-city violence in Boston are more than three times as likely to be diagnosed with asthma. In New York City, 50 percent of children entering a homeless shelter during the severe winter of 2004 were diagnosed with asthma. Infants born to mothers under stress are 60 percent more likely to wheeze in their first year of life. Mothers of asthmatic children have more marital problems and higher divorce rates.

Stress may increase our susceptibility to viral infections and bronchial reactivity. In cases where stress plays a major role in asthma, relaxation and biofeedback techniques may be helpful. Hypnotic suggestion may also benefit asthma. Other approaches that have been studied include behavior modification, verbal desensitization, and keeping a daily journal. Formal psychotherapy is rarely indicated in asthma, however, unless there is an independent psychiatric problem. Psychoactive drugs are sometimes required to treat associated anxiety or panic attacks or depression. When psychotropic drugs are utilized, it may be necessary to adjust doses of asthma drugs, as beta-agonists and theophylline may accentuate anxiety and the cortisone drugs can induce mood changes.

Non-Adherence or Non-Compliance

Dr. Robert Strunk notes that stress and emotional issues worsen asthma when they interfere with compliance and the proper use of medications.

Only one in every four people who suffer from asthma take their medications on a near-daily basis. Fifty to ninety percent of all people given a simple course of oral penicillin for a strep throat infection fail to complete their therapy. In ten pediatric adherence studies, medication compliance averaged 48 percent. In one asthma study, only 70 percent of new asthma prescriptions written by general practitioners were actually filled by the pharmacy. Nearly one-third of the people in the study did not use their beta-agonists as prescribed. They ignored their peak flow meters and did not carry their EpiPens as recommended.

ARE YOU COMPLIANT?

Dr. Bruce Bender, Professor of Psychiatry at National Jewish Hospital, defines adherence or compliance as the extent to which a patient follows a reasonable treatment plan that has been prescribed by a qualified caregiver. Bender has described three types of patients. The first is the compliant patient who takes most of his medications most of the time. The second patient uses medications when asthma symptoms flare. The third patient takes less than 25 percent of her medications.

Non-adherence leads to more emergency room visits and hospital-izations and has been closely linked to asthma deaths. For whatever reason, the sickest people are often the most non-adherent. Some of the reasons for non-adherence include denial of the disease, no imme-diate effects when treatment is stopped, the expense of asthma drugs, and too complex a treatment program.

Non-adherence is a very common problem in adolescents with asthma, as peer pressure leads to a total disregard of asthma medica-tions. Inhaler overuse is the biggest threat in this age group.

Surprisingly, non-adherence is less of a problem in elderly adults; however, non-compliance in this age group is usually due to a failing memory, a confusing medication schedule, and the high costs of asthma drugs. Patient distrust of their caregiver is another reason for non-adherence. It is human nature not to take a drug if you are feeling well.

The patient or family needs to take an active role in managing their asthma. They should do the following:

- Keep a written list of medications.
- Learn the names of their asthma medicines.
- Keep a diary of asthma symptoms and medication use.
- Keep accurate pill counts.
- Review instructions on proper inhaler usage.
- Read educational material on asthma.
- Enroll in asthma self-help programs.

The Role of Anxiety and Depression

Depression may play a major role in asthma. Depressed mothers liv-ing in inner cities are more likely to bring their asthmatic child to the emergency room. The two most common psychological reactions to asthma are anxiety and depression. The unpredictable nature of asthma may cause a sense of losing control over bodily functions. This leads to a feeling of vulnerability, fear, and anxiety. Because breathing is so central to survival, the loss of respiratory function is threatening. Anxiety may also be worsened by reactions of friends and family members. Depression is a reaction to the helplessness and loss of self-esteem caused by asthma. The major signs of severe depression are sleep disturbance, loss of interest in usual activities, loss of appetite, crying spells, and difficulty concentrating. When the level of the depression is moderate, antidepressant drugs may help. Relaxation techniques, deep breathing, understanding the effects of anxiety on breathing, and learning to differentiate the effects of asthma on breathing are all important steps to combat depression. Severe depression requires a consultation with a psychologist or psychiatrist.

CHAPTER TWENTY-FIVE

Mastering Your Tools: Inhalers, Asthma Spacers, Home Nebulizers, and Peak Flow Meters

To keep your asthma under control, you need to learn how to use your tools. Here's the lowdown on the most important tools you'll use.

Proper Inhaler Use

A pocket inhaler delivers a measured amount of drug and produces excellent results when people follow instructions and prescribed dosing intervals. Unfortunately, many asthmatics either overuse their inhalers or do not follow instructions. Some people have never been properly taught how to use an inhaler. The most common patient errors are improper activation of the inhaler, not waiting between inhalations, forgetting to shake the inhaler, and not keeping the inhaler clean. The basic steps for proper inhaler use are outlined here.

- Shake the inhaler thoroughly.
- Breathe out slowly and steadily.

- Hold your breath six to ten seconds.
- Hold the inhaler two inches from your mouth.
- Tilt your head up and activate the inhaler.
- Breathe in very slowly and as deeply as possible.
- Breathe out slowly and steadily.
- Wait one minute between sprays.

Dry Powder Inhalers

Non-pressurized or dry powder inhalers (DPIs) are becoming more widely available and will eventually replace the freon-propelled inhalers. Many people find them easier to use. As these devices are breath-activated, people do not need to coordinate breathing in with the discharge of the aerosol. DPIs reduce the incidence of the voice huskiness or throat irritation caused by the propellants present in some MDIs. The DPIs have some disadvantages. In contrast to the MDI, they require a stronger inspiration to maximize drug delivery. They may be less effective in severe asthma or unsuitable for children younger than four years of age. A DPI is an acceptable alternative to the MDI, provided the patient can generate enough of a deep breath to inhale the powder. Many newer DPIs come with a dose-counting device that lets you know when the inhaler is running low.

The Need for Caution

Three reports highlight the need for caution when using an MDI. One case describes a twenty-five-year-old male who awoke with an acute asthma attack in the middle of the night and reached for his bedside MDI. In the process of doing so, he did not remove the inhaler cap and subsequently inhaled it, which resulted in obstruction of his upper airway. Fortunately, he was able to remove the cap from his upper airway on his own. The only adverse reaction he experienced was pain and hoarseness that persisted for two months. The second report involved a forty-six-year-old man who developed acute respiratory distress after using his MDI. He kept his uncapped MDI together with some loose change in his pants pocket. After he developed choking and coughing, a chest X-ray showed a coin in his bronchial tube that was subsequently removed by passing a tube down his windpipe. The third case involved a nineteen-year-old woman who had acute throat pain and difficulty breathing after using her metered-dose inhaler. This patient was in the habit of storing her tetracycline capsules in the mouthpiece. Shortly after using her inhaler, she began coughing and successfully coughed up the tetracycline capsule fragment. If you suffer from asthma, these cases should alert you to the potential hazards of MDIs. You should check the inhaler mouthpiece before use and cap the device after using.

Asthma Spacers

One of the more subtle advances in asthma therapy has been the development of inhaler devices, known as spacers or holding chambers, that make it easier to use the MDIs. These inhaler aids allow young children, uncoordinated people, and elderly asthmatics with arthritis to use their inhalers more effectively. Spacers allow more aerosol spray to penetrate deeper into the lungs of people who cannot coordinate the release of the spray with taking a deep breath. The big advantage of the spacing devices is that large particles of the medications are deposited on the sides of the tube, leaving only the smaller particles, which are more easily inhaled into the lung. Fewer large particles end up being deposited in the mouth or the back of the throat. Using inhalers with spacers is the most versatile and cost-effective way to deliver an aerosol. Provided it is used properly, a large-volume spacer may double the amount of the drug that is delivered to the lung in comparison with what a well-trained patient can achieve using an MDI. The addition of a spacer to the MDI limits the amount of medication deposited in the mouth and throat, and also reduces the systemic absorption of the inhaled drug.

Home Nebulizers

People with mild or moderate asthma usually do quite well with a DPI, or an MDI with a spacer. Some people with more severe asthma need home compressors to administer aerosol medications at home. Devices like the DeVilbis Nebulizer, Pulmo-Aide, or the portable DuraNeb 2000 are actually mini-versions of the equipment used in the hospital by respiratory therapists. Medication added to a nebulizer is inhaled via a facemask or a mouthpiece. New versions of nebulizers are very portable, and can be powered by small batteries or automobile cigarette lighters. The best candidates for nebulizers are infants and young children and elderly asthmatics who have difficulty with hand-held metered dose inhalers and cannot grasp the concepts of the MDIs even when spacers are used. The availability of unit dose packs for cromolyn (Intal), albuterol, and inhaled cortisone drugs has improved the nebulizer's overall effectiveness and ease of use. Some of my patients and families who prefer to use the DPIs or MDIs and spacers for routine daily medications only use nebulized drugs in acute attacks that do not respond to the hand-held inhalers.

Peak Flow Meters

Lung function or breathing tests are essential yardsticks in asthma diagnosis and management. Breathing tests can be compared to monitoring blood pressure in people with hypertension and blood sugar levels in diabetics. What is the peak expiratory flow rate, commonly called the peak flow? The peak flow is the amount of air one can exhale during a forced expiration after taking as full a breath as possible. Your peak flow rate can be measured by a relatively inexpensive portable device called a peak flow meter that measures the amount of air in liters (a liter is about a quart) you exhale per minute. People who have asthma relapses do not respond appropriately to the severity of their disease. The peak flow meter is a much more accurate instrument than the doctor's stethoscope in assessing the severity of an asthma relapse. The peak flow meter lets you know how well you are breathing. Peak flow meters come in various forms. There are approximately a dozen or so peak flow meters on the market. The typical device consists of a plastic or metal tube with a mouthpiece at one end. When you blow into the tube, a pointer moves along a scale and records how much and how fast you can blow air out of your lungs. When asthma is active, it is harder to exhale air, and the peak flow meter measures how much obstruction you have in your airways. The peak flow meter has many uses. It can assess the severity of acute or chronic asthma in the health-care provider's office or the emergency room. It is used before and after exercise to determine the presence or absence of exercise-induced asthma. It enables the patient or family to monitor asthma at home and whether to step up or step down asthma medications.

School personnel can use the peak flow meter to assess the student who experiences acute asthma in the gymnasium, playing field, or classroom. Lastly, it can detect what type of occupational exposures may be triggering asthma in the workplace. The peak flow meter is not a perfect instrument. It depends on the patient's ability and willingness to exhale as hard and as fast as possible. Also, it only measures function of the larger airways. Asthma affecting the smaller airways may go undetected by the peak flow meter. Patient and family education is of the utmost importance for the peak flow meter to be an effective instrument. People should be instructed how and when to use the peak flow meter, how to record peak flow rates, how to interpret the readings, and when to communicate with health-care providers.

Most adults and older children, occasionally even a three- or four-year-old, can be taught to generate a peak expiratory flow rate. As the peak flow rate is effort-dependent, people need to be coached to put forth their best effort. Peak flows can be recorded in a notebook, table, or graph. The NHLBI Guidelines recommend that peak flow decisions be based on the patient's "personal best," rather than using a percentage of a normal predicted value. Many people exhibit a wide variation between their morning and evening peak flow rate. A 20 percent swing in peak flow readings is a normal variation on a day-to-day basis. Those people whose peak flow rate drops in the morning are called "morning dippers." One's personal best peak flow rate often occurs in late afternoon or evening after maximum asthma therapy. Sometimes, a course of oral cortisone may be needed to establish one's personal best. I usually advise a new asthma patient to record their peak flow rate two to three times a day for two to three weeks after they have been placed on daily asthma medications. Once asthma stabilizes, the peak flow rates can be charted when warning signs occur or during an asthma relapse.

Doctors Guillermo Mendoza and Thomas Plaut strongly recommend using the Asthma Management Zone System, which uses a traffic light color code to develop an asthma action plan. Three zones based on the individual's personal best or predicted value are established. The green zone represents 80 percent or better of one's personal best—this signals a "go" or "all clear" signal that asthma is stable and routine treatment should continue. The yellow zone ranges from 50 to 80 percent of one's personal best, and indicates the need to proceed with caution. An acute relapse may be imminent, and you need to take action to get your asthma under control. A peak flow below 50 percent of the personal best signals a red or dangerous medical alert. Bronchodilator drugs should be administered and health-care providers should be notified if peak flow measurements do not immediately return to the yellow or green zone.

Some health-care providers advocate the use of peak flow meters for all asthmatics. Others feel the widespread use of peak flow meters is unnecessary, as it results in too intense a focus on asthma by the family or patient. I believe that the peak flow meter should be part of any asthma education program, but the effectiveness of the instrument ultimately depends on patient compliance. Retrospective studies on diabetics asked to measure their blood sugar at home have shown a high rate of non-compliance even among well-educated diabetics and their families. Similar problems with compliance occur with the use of the peak flow meter. Nearly half of the patients I see during an asthma relapse have not used a peak flow meter prior to coming to the emergency room or my office. I prescribe peak flow meters to every patient with persistent asthma who requires daily asthma medications. I do not divide all of my patients into green, yellow, and red zones. I prefer to use this approach in people with more moderate to severe unstable asthma. I also utilize peak flow meters to determine the presence or absence of occupational and exercise-induced asthma. Furthermore, the peak flow meter allows the on-call doctor to make a more objective analysis of asthma relapses by phone during the evening or on weekends. I do not think peak flow meters should be routinely utilized in people with mild asthma, as such use could potentially cause social hang-ups or emotional dysfunction similar to those seen in people with hypertension who monitor their own blood pressure on a daily basis.

In summary, the peak flow meter is a vital component of the management of persistent asthma, and it should be used in combination with education programs that stress appropriate use of medications, recognizing the early warning signs of relapsing asthma and implementing appropriate environmental controls. The peak flow meter should not replace spirometry or lung-function testing in a clinic or medical office as a way to assess people with moderate to severe asthma. Several studies have shown that the peak flow meter reading may be normal when the more accurate method of following asthma, the FEV1 (or one-second vital capacity), is profoundly depressed.

RESOURCES

Asthma Education Programs

Most asthma education programs developed for children share several common elements. They provide families with a series of learning opportunities—typically four to eight sessions lasting an hour—so that families can fully explore all aspects of managing childhood asthma. Programs provide the opportunity for families to learn new information, acquire and practice new skills, and review their experience in applying these skills in the home situation. Most of these programs review basic asthma mechanisms, asthma symptoms, environmental controls, and proper use of asthma medications. These programs encourage families to develop an active partnership with their care providers.

Most adult education models consist of single sessions to review educational materials like video and audiotapes or printed booklets. Another type of adult program involves efforts to improve asthma management through special asthma clinics or asthma centers where more intensive medical management is coupled with asthma education. A review of adult programs suggests that brief patient education programs may lead to gains in asthma knowledge. I suggest you contact the local chapters of the American Lung Association (ALA) or the Asthma and Allergy Foundation of America (AAFA) to learn about ongoing education programs in your area.

The Asthma and Allergy Foundation of America

The Asthma and Allergy Foundation of America, or AAFA, is a national, nonprofit, patient organization dedicated to improving the quality of life for people with asthma and their caregivers. AAFA provides practical information, community-based services, educational programs, support, and referrals through a national network of chapters and educational support groups. AAFA is the only asthma and allergy patient advocacy organization that sponsors research toward identifying better treatments and a cure for asthma and allergic diseases. AAFA's programs are designed to improve the quality of life and care for people with asthma and allergies in communities across the country.

AAFA's advocacy and outreach efforts have played an integral role in establishing national guidelines for the diagnosis and management of asthma and allergies; setting national standards to improve quality care for asthma sufferers; obtaining federal funding for asthma prevention programs; and strengthening laws that protect patient rights. To locate an AAFA chapter in your area, contact AAFA at 1233 20th St. NW, Suite 402, Washington, DC 20036; 1-800-7-ASTHMA, 202-466-7643; or visit their Web site at www.aafa.org

Allergy and Asthma Network Mothers of Asthmatics

In 1985, Nancy Sander, a mother of a child with asthma, founded the Allergy and Asthma Network—Mothers of Asthmatics known as AANMA. AANMA is committed to eliminating suffering and death due to asthma and allergies through education, advocacy, and community outreach and research programs. AANMA offers original books, videos, and pamphlets that are carefully reviewed by medical experts. It provides discounts for allergy and asthma products like peak flow meters or nebulizers. AANMA depends on membership support for its programs and publications. A donation of any amount brings you a year of award-winning publications, up-to-the-minute news, and research developments.

Contact AANMA at 2751 Prosperity Ave., Suite 150, Fairfax, VA, 22031; 800-878-4403. To view or download their resources, visit their Web site at www.aanma.org

The American Academy of Allergy, Asthma and Immunology

The American Academy of Allergy, Asthma and Immunology, or AAAAI, is a membership organization of over four thousand practicing physicians, academicians, and researchers from the United States and forty-two foreign countries. AAAAI fosters new advances and education in the field of asthma, allergy, and immunology and promotes research and professional competence in the field of medicine. AAAAI's Web site (www.aaaai.org) offers pollen counts, a listing of asthma camps, and a physician referral guide. *Asthma and Allergy Advocate* is an informative newsletter published by the American Academy of Allergy, Asthma and Immunology that offers practical information and health tips for asthma and allergy sufferers. To obtain it, call 414-272-6071, or write the AAAAI at 611 East Wells St., Milwaukee, WI 53202.

The American College of Allergy, Asthma and Immunology

The American College of Allergy, Asthma and Immunology, or ACAAI, is an organization of three thousand doctors dedicated to educating physicians and improving patient care by addressing the needs of practicing physicians and specialists in the field of asthma and allergy. ACAAI encourages research and maintains the skills of its members by sponsoring educational programs and scientific publications. For additional information, contact ACAAI at 85 Algonquin Road, Suite 550, Arlington Heights, IL 60005; 847-427-1200, or visit their Web site at www.allergy.mcg.edu

The American Lung Association

The American Lung Association, or ALA, has produced a broad range of informative literature for sufferers of all types of lung diseases, including asthma. ALA sponsors public information programs, anti-smoking programs, and camps for children with asthma. The Web site also provides the latest news and tips about asthma and information about your local lung association. To contact the ALA, call or write the national office, 1740 Broadway, New York, NY 10010-4374; 212-315-8700, or consult your local phonebook to find the ALA chapter nearest you. For more information, you can visit the ALA Web site at www.lungusa.org. ALA has opened a new service called Ask Us at their Web site. They will answers questions on all lung diseases via e-mail within twenty-four hours.

The National Institute of Allergy and Infectious Diseases

The National Institute of Allergy and Infectious Diseases (NIAID) is a division of the National Institutes of Health (NIH), which conducts broad-based research training programs dealing with the causes, prevention, control, and treatment of all allergic diseases. NIAID publishes several informative pamphlets for people with asthma. These materials can be obtained by contacting NIAID at 9000 Rockville Pike, Bethesda, MD 20205; 301-496-5717, or by visiting their Web site at www.niaid.nih.gov/default.htm

Global Allergy Information Network (GAIN)

The Global Allergy Information Network, or GAIN, was launched by the World Allergy Organization in September 2000 during their annual Congress in Sydney, Australia. GAIN aims to be the premier Internet Web site specializing in allergic disorders. Its intended audience includes both professional and lay people. A key feature of the Web site is a series of links to helpful Web sites around the world. Each month a new topic in allergy and asthma will be reviewed. Visit GAIN's Web site at www.worldallergy.org and register for the GAIN e-newsletter, which will alert you when new features and topics are added to the Web site.

Asthma Education Program

The Asthma Education Program, sponsored by the National Heart, Lung, and Blood Institute, has developed a reading and resource list for people with asthma and their families. They have published *Check Your Asthma IQ* and *Managing Asthma: A Guide for Schools*, as well as several other pamphlets on asthma. Their publication list can be obtained by writing to them at P.O. Box 30105, Bethesda, MD 20824-0105, 301-951-3260 or by visiting their Web site at www.nhlbi.nih.gov/index.htm

Asthma and Allergy Publications

Asthma Magazine is an outstanding asthma publication edited by Rachel Butler. *Asthma Magazine* strives to promote public education and create a partnership between the patient, physician, and other health-care professionals through education and awareness. Published five times a year by Mosby. To order *Asthma Magazine,* call 800-654-2452.

Allergies and Asthma for Dummies by William Berger, M.D. (IDG Worldwide Inc., 2004) is an interesting, motivating, and amusing book written by my good friend Dr. Bill Berger. This easy-to-read text covers asthma, hay fever, food reactions, and more. It's a valuable addition to one's allergy-asthma library.

Asthma Guide for People of All Ages by Thomas Plaut, M.D., includes information on medication and how to handle a variety of asthma symptoms. Dr. Plaut has also written *One Minute Asthma,* a concise pamphlet highlighting the principles of asthma therapy, and *Children with Asthma: A Manual for Parents,* an informative book for the parents of asthmatic children. These publications are available from Pedi Press, Inc., 125 Redgate Lane, Amherst, MA 01002. *Cooking for the Allergic Child* by Judy Moyer is an informative cookbook with over three hundred recipes, nutritional facts, and a fine resource section. Order through your bookstore or send $15.95 to Allergy Control Products, 89 Danbury Road, Ridgefield, CT 06877.

Understanding Asthma (University Press of Mississippi, Jackson, Mississippi) was written by my friend and scholarly colleague Phil Lieberman, M.D. This book provides a comprehensive review of how asthma affects the lungs. The section on immunology is well written and illustrated. Lieberman gives thoughtful insight into current research and future asthma therapies.

Guide to Your Children's Allergies and Asthma, edited by Michael Welch, M.D., published by Villard Books, is the latest in a series of parenting books from the American Academy of Pediatrics. A good resource book for parents who want up-to-date information on their child's allergies or asthma.

My House Is Killing Me! The Home Guide for Families with Allergies and Asthma, written by home inspector and science teacher Jeffrey May (Johns Hopkins University Press), is a very readable and informative book that takes the reader through the home on a room-by-room basis. May details how to identify and remove asthma and allergy triggers. Available at bookstores or at www.jhupbooks.com

Asthma Treatment Centers

In the late 1920s, Dr. Murray Peshkin admitted a group of severely ill asthmatic children to New York's Mount Sinai Hospital. Much to Dr. Peshkin's surprise, many children improved dramatically without specific treatment. It was obvious that an unstable home environment and family stress played a major role in asthma, and when children were removed from the parental home, they were able to overcome their asthma. Dr. Peshkin appropriately coined the term "parentectomy." This innovative program, which eventually moved to the more favorable climate of Denver, Colorado, led to the establishment of the world's leading asthma-allergy research center, now known as National Jewish Hospital. This center and others like it became residential treatment facilities for the care of children with severe asthma. Children were admitted to such centers for several weeks or months. Due to changes in the economics of medical care, virtually all of these programs have either closed or have converted to short-term treatment facilities. At National Jewish Hospital, the outdated approach that required a hospital stay of several weeks or months has been replaced by a new program called Time Out for Asthma. For additional information, call 1-800-NJC-9555, or visit their Web site, www.nationaljewish.org

Asthma Summer Camps

Another very successful educational approach for asthmatic children is the asthma summer camp. Many camps for asthmatic children have been established throughout the United States. Most are modeled after Camp Bronco Junction in Redhouse, West Virginia, which was founded by Dr. Merle Scherr, the pioneer of asthma summer camps. The American Lung Association sponsors most of these asthma camps. At last count there were eighty camps, serving 4,500 kids each summer. Programs vary from day camps to two-week overnight camps. Most camps have well-structured programs that stress self-help and basic asthma education. All approved camps have good medical supervision. While it may cost $350 to $400 per week for an overnight camp, the ALA or the camp sponsor will often pick up the tab for families who cannot afford the camp fee.

Contact your local chapter of the American Lung Association or the Asthma and Allergy Foundation of America to locate the nearest asthma summer camp in your area.

Employee Education Programs

Employers are now demanding improved quality of care and cost efficiencies through disease-management programs. The demands of employers are due in large part to the development of managed-care programs. Purchasers of health care are urging their insurers to implement asthma-management programs. When you consider that asthma costs American employers $4 billion a year, it is no surprise that many corporations have implemented asthma-education programs. Such programs are aimed at reducing emergency room visits, asthma hospitalizations, and work absenteeism. Most of these employer programs that were started in the early 1990s have shown a dramatic reduction in the costs of asthma care and improved quality of life for the participants.

Web Sites for Asthma Education

Health-care providers or interested consumers who want to learn about the most up-to-date diagnostic and treatment protocols for asthma can now access almost all the medical literature on asthma. One new Web site, called the Asthma Management Model System or AMMS, was designed by the NHLBI's National Asthma Education and Prevention Program (NAEPP). This wide-ranging system will search major scientific databases from MEDLINE, CRISP, and CORDIS, as well as documents from the CDC and the FDA. This AMMS Web site can be accessed via the NHLBI home page at www.nhlbi.nih.gov

National Allergy Bureau

The National Allergy Bureau, or NAB, is the leading source for pollen and spore count information in the United States. The AAAAI and ACAAI have joined forces to promote this valuable network. It serves as a public service to Americans who are concerned about allergens in their environment. NAB keeps people informed about aeroallergens in their environment and enables them to make proper decisions regarding medication use and environmental controls. For more information regarding NAB, contact the AAAAI at 414-272-6071 or visit their Web site at www.aaaai.org/nab.

Asthma and Allergy Supply Companies

The companies listed below all provide a wide range of allergy and asthma products including allergen barriers, cleaning supplies, air cleaners, respiratory products, and educational materials required to institute proper environmental controls in your home. Very few, if any, retail stores offer the quality of material and pricing available through these mail order houses. Most, if not all, of these companies have attractive brochures and Web sites that display their prices and products.

Allergy Etc: A one-stop source for allergy and environmental products. Their full line of products is listed in their award-winning Web site. 800-804-6022; www.allergyetc.com

Allergy Asthma Technology LTD.: 8224 Leigh Avenue, Morton Grove, IL. Offers quality products for asthma and allergy care and environmental controls. Colorful and complete brochure. 800-621-5545; Fax 847-966-3068; www.allergyasthmatech.com

Allergy Control Products: 96 Danbury Road, Ridgefield, CT 06877. 800-422-3878; Fax 203-431-8963. An eighteen-year-old company with a proven line of allergen-avoidance products designed to reduce allergen exposure in the home. www.allergycontrol.com

Allergy Direct: 2020 SW Fourth Avenue, Suite 750, Portland, OR 97201; 877-283-2323; www.allergydirect.com. Offers a wide selection of name-brand, physician-approved products and educational materials.

Allergy Free: 6835 Flanders Drive #500, San Diego, CA 95746; 916-789-4165; Fax 916-789-4159. Manufactures Aller-Pure Gold electrostatic filters. They also provide a complete line of allergen-avoidance products.

National Allergy Supply: 1620 Satellite Blvd., Suite D, P.O. Box 1658, Duluth, GA 30096; well-established company that offers full line of allergen-avoidance products. Offers new membrane-free encasements for bedding materials. 800-522-1448; www.nationalallergy.com

Allergy Solutions, Inc.: 7 Crozerville Road, Aston, PA 19014; 800-491-4300; Fax 484-840-0366; www.allergysolution.com. A complete source of environmental control, allergen avoidance and asthma management products.

Mission Allergy: 28 Hawleyville Road, Hawleyville, CT 06440; 203-364-1570; Fax 203-426-5607; www.missionallergy.com. Manufactures high-quality microfiber pillow and mattress encasings. Offers Self-Help Guide for accurate information on allergen avoidance.

INDEX